Perspectives in Environmental Health : Vector & Water Borne Diseases

Edited by:

Dr. Amit Krishna De

Dr. Aniruddha Mukhopadhyay

Originals

(an imprint of Low Price Publications)

Delhi-110052

Distributed by
D.K. Publishers Distributors (P) Ltd.
4834/24, Ansari Road, Darya Ganj,
New Delhi-110002
Phones: 51562573, 51562575, 51562577,
e-mail: dkpd@del3.vsnl.net.in
visit us at: www.dkpd.com

ISBN 81-88629-29-4

Published by
Originals
(an imprint of Low Price Publications)
A-6, Nimri Commercial Centre,
Near Ashok Vihar Phase-IV,
Delhi-110052
Phones: 27452453
e-mail: lpp@nde.vsnl.net.in
visit us at: www.lppindia.com

Printed at
D K Fine Art Press P Ltd.
Delhi-110052

PRINTED IN INDIA

Contents

Section II - Water Borne Diseases

Foreword

The publication of the book *Perspectives In Environmental Health: Vector & Water Borne Diseases* brings forth a concise collection of different health problems faced in our communities together with suitable practices to protect the common public; thereby allowing a deep sense of awareness about our environment, to grow within us.

The agents of transmission referred to as "vectors" play a significant role in dissemination of a wide variety of infections. The disease burden from spread of malarial parasites is a staggering one and warrants active and effective control measures to protect the susceptible population across our country. It is of utmost importance to educate our countrymen and this book presents a very useful collection of facts that should arouse any reader to "believe" that the time is ripe now to harness our resources to effectively combat vector borne inflections in the environment, leading to safer habitats which could save our children and youth who constitute the future "wealth" of our country.

The requirement for safe potable water is a national issue; however unknown instances of faecal oral transmission of a variety of bacterial and viral infections through water remains our serious concern. The spread of deadly diseases like cholera can quickly grow into epidemic proportions in any neighbourhood where the infectious strain has entered and polluted the water. This water is soon unknowingly "taken" by people, and in our densely populated country, large numbers become affected within a very short time, as they commonly share the infection. The role of rotavirus or cholera in acute watery diarrohoea is a deplorable one and a completely safe vaccine is still being eagerly sought, for the past few decades. As one browses through the chapters in this book the message is very clear that adoption of hygienic practices is very essential and safeguarding the neighbourhood will protect the unwanted spread of diseases, making our livelihood a better one in the near future.

I hope the readers will immensely benefit from reading this book and hereafter enjoy a richer, healthier life in a safer environment.

Prof. Manish Chakraborty
Former Director of School of Tropical Medicine, Kolkata
and Honorary Director, ICMR Virus Unit, Kolkata

Preface

The World Health Organisation (WHO) has provided a wholesome definition of health - "Health is a state of complete physical, mental and social well-being and not merely the absence of disease of infirmity". WHO adds, "The maintenance and improvement of health should be at the centre of concern about environment and development. Yet health rarely receives high priority in environmental policies and developmental plans, rarely figures as an important item in environmental and developmental programmes, despite the fact that the quality of the environment and the nature of development and major determinants of health".

Following will justify the above statement:

(i) Two thousand million people are at risk from waterborne and foodborne diarrhoeal diseases, which are the main cause of nearly four million deaths each year.

(ii) Over a million people die from malaria each year and 276 millions are infected.

(iii) Hundreds of millions suffer from intestinal parasitic infections.

(iv) 90 million people are infected each year with filariasis.

(v) 30-60 million people are infected each year with dengue fever.

(vi) Nearly half of the total world population suffers from diseases associated with insufficient and contaminated water, mostly the poor and virtually all in developing countries.

India, a developing third world country is unique considering its geography, climate flora, and fauna and peoples diversity. It has got a vast water resource, both marine and freshwater, with large agricultural lands and moderate forest cover but the alarmingly increasing trend of population level has caused a panic with irrational use of the environmental wealth. In reality, the environment has given us much to satisfy our needs but not much to satisfy our greed. In recent years, several issues concerning environment have come up, one of such is environment health.

Environmental health is a buzzword these days. In general, vectorborne and waterborne diseases are a global problem, though it is particularly prevalent in the tropical countries. In a country like India it draws a special attention considering its population size (a) Vector Biology and Ecology (b) Clinico-Epidemiology (c) Chemotherapy (d) Parasitology (e) Microbiology (f) Molecular Biology and Genetics (g) Immunology (h) Environmental Management (i) Socio-Economics (j) Public health hygiene and Awareness, have been accomodated in the book.

Most of the selected papers were presented at the symposium held at Bose Institute in Decemeber 1999. Rest of the papers are invited from renowned experts from different Research Institutes and Universities in West Bengal. It won't be out of place to mention here that the content of the book will attract a large cross section of people ranging from different academic, research and administrative disciplines including Medical and general bioscience students (e.g. Microbiology, Biotechnology, Zoology, Parasitology, Biochemistry, Environmental Science, Immunology, Molecular Biology etc.), Researchers, Medical Pracitioners, Public Health Workers, NGO's, Environmental Engineers, City Planners, Panchayat and Municipal workers and Ecological Activities.

There are two sections in the book. Section-I covers the Vectorborne and Section-II, the waterborne diseases. Finally, this book focuses on the present perspective of the environment health problems and shows a new direction and approach towards a solution.

Dr Aniruddha Mukhopadhyay
Dr Amit Krishna De

Section I

Vector Borne Diseases

Chapter - 1

Vectors and Vector-borne Diseases

** Buddhadeb Manna*

Abstract

Arthropods like mosquitoes, fleas, flies, ticks and mites are major vectors for viral, bacterial, protozoal and hilminth transmission, although some infections are transmitted by other invertebrates, even some vertebrates. Mosquitoes transmit about 90 viruses other than malarias and filarias. Flies spread 20 viral, bacterial, protozoan and helminth infections. Other nonbiting flies transmit trachoma, yaws and tropical ulcers. Cockroaches spread faecal pathogens mechanically. Ticks and mites transmit many bacterial and protozoal diseases and also act as intermediate host for many helminth parasites.

Introduction

The knowledge of vectors and vector-borne diseases is of very much importance to control different epidemics, epizootics and zoonotic diseases (Beaver *et al.*, 1984; Cheng, 1986; Roberts and Janovy, 1996; Harwood and James, 1979). The veterinarians, live-stock inspectors and their family, butchers, slaughter men, handlers of meat, milk, eggs, hides, fur etc, wild life workers, foresters, hunters, surveyors, explorers, tourists, zoo garden employees, wild-life park employees and visitors, pet or wild animal dealers, animal autopsy performers, laboratory animal handlers, veterinary public health workers, disaster victims, refugees, and pilgrimage participants are the group of people specially at risk for contact of such diseases (Chakraborty, 1991). Now we are in a position to understand the transmission cycle of many of the diseases of man and other nonhuman animals. Vectors play a vital role in maintaining the continuity of the disease process and acting also as the reservoir hosts. The knowledge of biology of vectors will help to control the epidemic and epizootic diseases. Most of the eradication or control programmes of the diseases fail due to

* Department of Zoology, University of Calcutta, Kolkata-700019

incomplete knowledge of vector biology and its inter-relation to the disease processes prevailing in nature.

Vectors

The word **Vector** is used by the epidemiologists to indicate a live animal that transmit an infectious agents from one host to another. The majority of vectors are arthropods such as mosquitoes, fleas, flies, and ticks, although larger animals can also spread infections. For example rabies is transmitted by mammals, psittacosis is transmitted by birds, salmonellosis by lower vertebrates etc (Cheng, 1986; Palmer *et al.*, 1998).

Vector classified

Vectors are placed into one of two categories, biological and mechanical, depending upon the animal's relationship with the infection agents.

A biological vector actively participates in a pathogen's life cycle, serving as a site in which it can multiply or complete its life cycle. A biological vector communicates the infectious agent to the human or other hosts by biting, aerosal formation or touch. In the case of biting vectors the animals can (i) inject infected saliva into the blood like mosquitoes, (ii) defeacate around the bite wound, like the fleas, or (iii) regurgitate blood into the wound, like tsetse fly.

The mechanical vectors are not necessary to the life cycle of an infectious agent and merely transport it without being infected. The external body parts of these animals become contaminated when they come into physical contact with a source of pathogens. The agent is subsequently transferred to humans indirectly by an intermediate such as food or, occasionally, by direct contact, as in eye infection.

House flies have habits that suit them to the role of mechanical vector. Their mouth parts are adapted for feeding on decaying garbage and faeces, and while they are feeding their feet and mouth parts can easily become contaminated. They also regurgitate juices onto food to soften and digest it. Flies spread more than 20 bacterial, viral, protozoans and worm infections. Other nonbiting flies transmit tropical ulcers, yaws, trachoma. Cockroaches, which have similar habit play a role in the mechanical transmission of faecal pathogens as well as contributing to allergy attacks in asthmatic children.

Many vectors and animal reservoirs spread their own infections to human. Each pathogen has its own peculiarities of lifestyle within the vector. Pathogen like *Yersinia pestis* shows propagative transmission mode. Pathogen multiplies in the insect host but undergoes no developmental changes. Large number of pathogens leaving the flea are essentially the same as those ingested. Some pathogens and parasites like trypanosomes, malarial parasites etc. show cyclopropagative transmission. They not only multiplies in the insect body but also changes its form in some manner. In case of helminths like filarial worm cyclodevelopmental transmission occurs. Here pathogen undergoes a developmental transformation in the vector but does not multiply.

Vector borne diseases

The most important vectors are insects like mosquitoes, flies, fleas, ticks and mites and other invertebrates as well as some vertebrates.

1. Mosquitoes as vectors

The mosquito is the number one vector for many diseases. The most important and largest genera transmitting diseases are *Culex, Aedes, Anopheles, Mansonia, Coquilletida* and *Culiseta* (Harwood and James, 1979).

A. Viral transmission

Berge (1975) catalogued approximately 90 viruses isolated from mosquitoes. Only few are mentioned below.

a. *Yellow fever* (Flavivirus). *Aedes aegypti* is recognised as the vector of yellow fever virus in urban area. The mosquito gets virus during patient's blood feeding. The period of incubation in mosquito is 12 days or more and the mosquito remains infective throughout the rest of life, 200 days or more. In man incubation period is about 3-4 days. Sudden attack of fever with headache, backache, vomiting, dark vomit after 2-3 days, gradual yellowing of mucous membrane and skin are the symptoms of the disease. In the jungle *Aedes aegypti* is absent hence the vector of the disease is *Haemagogus* sp., which breeds in tree-holes, act as reservoir of the virus and transfer it to monkeys and to occasional travellers who pass through the jungle. The traveller so infected passes on the virus to *Aedes aegypti* when arrives in the city and starts its cycle in urban area. However, the disease occurrence is absent in India.

b. *Dengue fever* (Flavivirus) or Break-bone fever. *Aedes aegypti* is the vector in India, *A. albopictus* is the probable vector in Philippines. The incubation period of virus in mosquito is 8-14 days and thereafter the mosquito remains infective throughout life.

c. *Human and equine viral encephalitis.* Birds are the reservoir host and the cycle continue between man and animal. *Aedes, Culex, Anopheles, Mansonia* are the vector of this virus. Fever with nausea, vomiting accompanied with mental lapses, stiffening of neck, convulsion and paralysis are observed.

d. *Rift-valley fever. Aedes* spp are the vectors. Cattle, sheep etc. are also attacked. Abdominal discomfort along with pain in the joints and fever are the symptoms (Palmer *et al.*, 1998).

e. *West Nile disease.* This viral disease is transmitted by *Culex univittetus, C. antennatus, C. tritaeniorhynchus,* and *C. pipiens fatigans.*

f. *Fowl pox.* This virus is transmitted by *Aedes aegypti and A. stimulans.*

g. *Myxomatosis.* This virus disease of rabbits are transmitted by *Aedes scapularis,* and *A. aegypti.*

h. *Japanese B encephalitis.* The virus in India is transmitted by *Culex vishnui, C. pseudovishnui, C. tritaeniorhynchus.* Some species of *Anopheles* and *Mansonia* are also capable of transmission. It is a zoonotic. Headache, vomiting, diarrhoea, nausea, high fever, ocular disorientation, coma and convulsion are associated with the disease.

i. *Chikungunya fever.* In India *Aedes aegypti, Culex pipiens fatigans* are the vectors. Incubation period is 3-12 days. High fever with pain in joints and back are the symptoms. Monkey and Apes are the reservoir hosts.

B. Bacterial association

Aedes aegypti, A. crinifer, Psorophora, Culex scapularis, Anopheles albitarsis show positive for transfer of *Mycobacterium leprae* in experimental feeding on the leprosy patient.

C. Protozoan infections

Malaria is the most important mosquito-borne disease of man, monkey, and apes. The human malaria parasites include *Plasmodium vivax, P. falciparum, P. ovale,* and *P. malariae* are transmitted by various species of *Anopheles. P. simium* of howler monkeys of South America, *P. fieldi* of Malayan monkey, *P. simiovale* of *Macaca sinica* of Sri Lanka, *P. inui* of old world monkey, *P. shortti* of Bonnet monkey of Nicobar Islands, *P. hylobati* of Hylobates spp of South East Asia, *P. brasilianum* of New World monkeys along the course of Amazon river in Brazil, *P. cynomolgi of Macaca irus, P. berghei* of different sylvatic rats, *P. knowlesi of Macaca* spp and *Presbytis* sp. are all transmitted by different species of *Anopheles.*

P. gallinaceum and *P. relictum* are the bird malaria transmitted by *Aedes, Culex, Armigeres, Culiseta,* and *Anopheles* mosquitoes.

D. Helminth infections

The nematode parasites transmitted by mosquitoes are mostly related to the filarias. *Wuchereria bancrofti* transmitted by *Culex* spp. including *C. quinquefasciatus, Aedes* spp. *Mansonia* spp. and *Anopheles* spp., *Brugia malayi* is transmitted by *Culex pipiens quinquefasciatus, C.p. pallens, Aedes polynesiensis, A. togoi, Coquillettidia* spp., *Mansonia* spp., *Anopheles gambiae, A. funestus, A faranti, A. pyrcanus sinensis. Dirofilaria imitis* in dogs, cats, and wild carnivores are transmitted by *Culex pipiens, Aedes aegypti* and *Mansonia* spp.

2. ***Sand fly*** (*Phlebotomus* spp.)

a. *Viral infection.* A short duration (three days) viral fever during May to October is transmitted by *Phlebotomus papatasi.* Incubation period in the sand fly is 7-10 days.

b. *Carrion's disease or Bartonellosis. Phelobotomus verrucarum* transmits *Bartonella bacilliformis,* a rickettsian which parasitises the erythrocytes, endothelial cells of lymph glands and other organs of man and causes carrion's disease or "Oroya fever".

c. *Visceral leishmaniasis. Leishmania donovani* transmitted by sand flay *Phlebotomus argentipes* in India, *P. chinensis* in China, *P. perniciosus* in Mediterranean countries and *P. longipalpis* in Brazil cause kala azar or visceral leishmaniasis. In this disease the skin darkens, enlargement of spleen and liver and death in acute infection within 2-3 years occurs (Beaver *et al,* 1984).

d. *Cutaneous leishmaniasis.* The parasite *Leishmania tropica* transmitted by *Phlebotomus papatasi* and *P. sergenti* in India, Middle East, Congo and other countries cause Cutaneous leishmaniasis or Delhi boil. Incubation period is 8-21 days.

e. *Espundia or Mucocutaneous leishmaniasis.* The parasite *Leishmania braziliensis* transmitted by *Lutzmyia* sp in South and Central America cause Espundia disease. The parasite attacks the mucocutaneous junctions and destroy tissues including bones and cartilages.

3. *Culicoides* spp.

a. *Viral infection.* Virus disease like "*Blue tongue*" of sheep, *Horse sickness* of South America and *Fowl pox* of Japan are suspected to be transmitted by *Culicoides* spp.

b. *Malaria-like blood infection. Parahaemoproteus nettionis* a malaria-like blood parasite of duck and water fowl is transmitted by *Culicoides* sp. *Hepatocystis kochi,* a malaria-like blood parasite of monkeys in Africa is transmitted by *Culicoides adersi. Rayella* sp. a malaria-like parasite of flying squirrel (Dasgupta and Pal, 1976) in Darjeeling is transmitted by *Culicoides* sp.

c. *Filarial infection.* A human filaria *Dipetalonema (=Acanthocheilonema) perstans* in West Africa is transmitted by *Culicoides austeni* and *C. grahami. Mansonella ozzardi,* another filarial worm of man is transmitted by *Culicoides furens* in Central and South America.

4. *Simulid flies or Dimdam flies of North-East India*

Simulium damnosum in West Africa, *S.ochraceum* in Guatemala, transmit a filarial worm *Onchocerca volvulus* in man and *Ogutturosa* in cattle. The protozoan blood parasites of birds like *Leucocytozoon simondi* and *L. sakharoffi* and virus disease like Eastern equine encephalitis and vesicular stomatitis of certain birds, are transmitted by certain species of *Simulium.*

5. *Tabanus sp.*

Bacillus anthracis causing carbuncle in domestic animals and man are transmitted by *Tabanus* sp. *Pulmonary anthrax* may be caused simply by inhalation of spores. Ingestion of spores may also cause intestinal anthrax. *Tabanus striatus* may also cause sleeping sickness of cattle by transmitting *Trypanosoma brucei evansi* mechanically.

6. *Chrysops dimidiata*

Loa loa a filarial worm preferentially harbour in the anterior chamber of eye in some parts of Africa is transmitted by *Chrysops dimidiata* and *C. silacea.* The adult parasites also harbour in tongue, back, finger, breast and scrotum.

Chrysops discatis mechanically transmit *Francisella* (= *Pasteurella*) *tularensis,* causing tularemia in man, where fever with pain and lymph gland swellings develop.

7. *House flies*

The house fly *Musca* spp. mechanically transmits many viral, bacterial, protozoans and helminthic diseases.

It can transmit *Trachoma* virus affecting eyes of healthy man and *Bacillus anthracis* causing anthrax. *Mycobacterium tuberculi* causing tuberculosis, *Mycobacterium leprae,* causing leprosy, *Shigella dysentreriae* causing bacillary dysentery, *Vibrio cholerae* causing cholera, *Salmonella typhi,* the bacillus causing typhoid, *Treponema pertenue,* the spirochaete causing yaws, and *Helicobacter pylori,* a bacterium causing stomach ulcer. The cysts of *Entamoeba, Giardia,* causing protozoal dysentery, helminth eggs like *Enterobius, Ascaris, Trichuris, Ancylostoma, Taenia* etc. are also transmitted by house flies.

8. Glossina spp.

Glossina palpalis and *G. tachinoides* transmit *Trypanosoma brucei gambiense* causing sleeping sickness in man in Africa while *G. morsitans, G. swynertoni and G. pallidipes* transmit *T. brucei rhodesiense* the rhodesian form of trypanosomosis in man.

9. Fleas

Of the fleas *Xenopsylla cheopis* is very much medically important in transmitting dangerous disease like bubonic plague. Other species *Pulex irritans* is specific parasite of man, also may attack dogs and cats. *Ctenocephalids canis* is specific parasite of dog, *Ctenocephalids felis* is parasite of cat but both may attack man. *Spilopsyllus cuniculi* harbour in the ear of rabbits and other rodents. *Ceratophyllus gallinae* is a common flea of poultry which may attack man, and *Echidnophaga gallinacea* is parasite of fowls but may attack mammals. The fleas transmit the following diseases.

a. *Plague.* The bacillus *Yersinia* (=*Pasteurella*) *pestis* cause the epidemic bubonic plague of man, transmitted by the flea *Xenopsylla cheopis,* the rat flea. This flea acquire infection from the infected rat. After death of rat it jumps upto 18 cm and may bite man and thus man become infected. Wild rodents are reservoir of the disease.

b. *Murine typhus. Pulex irritans* another flea transmit *Rickettsia prowazeki* var *typhi* to man. Sometimes *Ctenocephalids canis* and *C. felis* also transmit the disease.

c. *Helminth infection.* The eggs of *Dipylidium caninum,* the common tape-worm of cats and dogs occurring in faecal matter of the host (Manna, 1996) are taken up by the larvae of *P. irritans, C. canis* and *C. felis* and develops cysticercus larvae. While leaking its body the dogs swallow such infected flea and thus infection is established. Similarly *Dipetalonema reconditum,* a filarial worm of dog in *C. canis* and *C. felis* gets entry.

10. Bug

a. *Kissing bug or Assassin bug. Panstrongylus* (=*Triatoma*) *megistus* in Brazil and adjoining countries of South America transmits *Schizotrỳpanum cruzi.* This starcorarian trypanosome caused Chagas' disease. While sucking blood this insect passes faecal matters with the infective forms of the trypanosome which enter into man through his soiled fingers with which he may touch his mucous membrane (Palmer *et al.*, 1998).

b. *Bed-bug. Cimex lectularius* and *C. hemipterus* (=*rotundatus*) common wingless blood sucking bed-bugs in India are considered as transmitter of many bacterial, viral and protozoal diseases but now established that it has nothing to do with the transmission process.

11. Sucking louse

These are obligatory ectoparasites in the hair of head and body parts. *Pediculus humanus capitis* and *P.h. corporis, Phthirus pubis,* the crab-louse or pubic louse are important vector for many diseases. The Typhus organism *Rickettsia prowazeki* var *prowazeki* is transmitted by both *P.h. capitis* and *P.h. corporis. Rickettsia prowazeki* var *typhi* causing *Murine typhus, R. wolhynica* (=*quintana*) causing Trench fever, the spirochaete *Bornelia recurrentis* causing relapsing fever, *Francisella* (= *Pasteurella*) *pestis* causing *Tularaemia* and *Yersinia pestis* causing plague are transmitted by these head and body louse.

12. Cockroaches

The cockroaches act as vector of hook worm *Necator americanus.* whipworm *Trichuris trichiura.* The pathogens isolated from cockroaches include cysts of *Entamoeba histolytica,* a large number of pathogens including *Mycobacterium leprae, Bacillus anthracis, Vibrio cholerae, Clostridium tetani, Giazdia intestinalis* and *Balantidium coli.*

13. Ticks

All ticks are blood sucker and most of them are vectors of many diseases. They remain hiding at day time in nest or in crevices. Ticks require blood meal prior to moulting from larval stage to nymphal stage and from later stage to adulthood. *Argas persicus* attacks fowl at night, transmit the spirochaete *Borrelia recurrentis* causing relapsing fever and the piroplasm *Aegyptianella pollurum. Ornithodorous* spp. transmit virus of African swine fever, a rickettsian *Coxiella burnetti* causing Queensland fever (Q-fever) of man and animals; *Leptospira icterohaemorrhagiae* causing Weil's disease (infectious jundice); *Francisella* (=*Pasteurella*) *tulerensis* causing tularaemia and *Borrelia duttoni* causing African relapsing fever (Beaver *et al.*, 1984).

Ixodes ricinus of cattle and sheeps transmit *Staphylococcus aureus* causing pyemia and a piroplasm *Babesia divergens* causing red-water fever. Adult *I. scapularis* prefers blood of white tailed deer and acquires spirochaete *Borrelia burgdorferi* and transmits to man causing Lyme disease characterised by juvenile rheumatoid.

Haemaphysalis sp., a three-host tick, parasitise, birds and mammals, transmits *Babesia major* and *B. bigemina, B. motasi,* to cattle and sheep, causing tick paralysis, complete respiratory and heart failure and also transmit rickettsial diseases including Q-fever.

Dermacentor spp are vector of *Babesia* of horses. Some species transmit *Anaplasma maginale* of cattle, *Dermacentroxenus rickettsi* causing Rocky mountain spotted fever in man, *Coxiella burnetti* causing Q-fever in man and also *Francisella* sp causing tularaemia in man.

Amblyomma spp transmit Rocky Mountain spotted fever, Q-fever, tularaemia and heart-water disease. *Boophilus* spp transmit *Anaplasma* and *Babesia. Rhipicephalus* spp are the vectors of *Theileria parva* causing East Coast fever of cattle, *Babesia bigemina,* Nairobi sheep disease, and good number of other microbes. *Kyasanur forest virus* are transmitted by *Haemaphysalis, Ixodes* and *Dermacentor* spp.

14. Mites

Demodex spp causes 'mange' lesion leading to *Staphylococcus* infection causing death of dogs, cats, cattle and horses (Basu, Chatterjee and Aich, 1985).

Sarcoptes scabiei cause scabies in man and mange in animals, live under the skin of mammals and birds. The disease spreads through infected clothing and infected animals like goat, sheep, pigs, cattle and dogs. *Ornithonyssus* spp parasitise poultry and wild birds and transmit rickettsians causing Q-fever, typhus, tularaemia, reckettsial pox and also cotton rat filariasis.

The larvae of *Trombicula akamushi* attack man and transmits *Rickettsia tsutsugamushi,* the causative organism of Asiatic scrub typhus to man and remains as carrier of the microbe through successive generations transovarially.

References

- Basu, A.K., Chatterjee, A.P. and Aich, A.C. (1985). Efficacy of Neguvon on Demodex infection in a heifer. *Indian J. Anim. Hlth.* **24(2)** : 155.
- Beaver, P.C., Jung, R.C. and Cupp, E.W. (1984). *Clinical Parasitology.* 9th ed. Lea & Febiger, Philadelphia.
- Berge, T.O. (ed.) (1975). *International catalogue of arboviruses including certain other viruses of vertebrates.* U.S. Dept. Health, Education, and Welfare, Publ. No. (CDC) 75-8301. Government Printing Office, Washington D.C.
- Chakraborty, M.S. (1991). Arboviral zoonoses. *Proceedings of the Seminar on zoonoses.* Edited by L.P. Dutta. Library and Documentation Division. Regional Medical Research Centre. N.E. Region (ICMR), Dibrugarh, Assam, pp. 12-16.
- Cheng, T.C. (1986). Introduction to parasitic insects. In "*General Parasitology*" by T.C. Cheng. 2nd ed. Academic Press. USA. pp. 614.
- Dasgupta, B. and Pal, N. (1976). Malarial Oocyst in *Culicoides* sp in Darjeeling. *Transactions of the Royal Society of Tropical Medicine and Hygiene.* **70:** 89-90
- Harwood, R.F. and James, M.T. (1979). "*Entomology in Human and Animal Health*" 7th ed. Macmillan, New York.
- Manna, B. (1996). Zoonosis and Zoonotic Parasites. In Zoology in *Modern times,* Proceedings of the first Refresher Course in Zoology, January 1-20, 1996. University of Calcutta. Academic Staff College. pp. 86-89.
- Palmer, S.R., Soulsby, L. and Simpson, D.I.H. (1998). *Zoonoses.* Oxford University Press Inc. New York.
- Roberts, L.S. and Janovy, Jr. J. (1996). *Foundations of Parasitology.* 5th ed. Times Mirror Higher Education Group. Inc. USA.

Chapter - 2

Recent Epidemiology and Control Activities of Malaria in West Bengal

** A. K. Mukhopadhyay*

Abstract

The history of control of malaria in India has seen tremendous successes as well as failures. It has been responsible for considerable degree of morbidity and mortality during pre-independence and continues its onslaught on the health and economy of the country including West Bengal in the early years of post independence of India. In early 1960s, malaria apparently disappeared from the country due to control activities by National Malaria Control Programme (1953), which later switched over to National Malaria Eradication Programme (1958), helped the country to recover in economic fronts. After initial stabilisation of the disease subsequent to the launching of Modified Plan of Operation (1977), there have been localised out break. Since 1994 onwards considerable degree of mortality, prompted the nation to review the current control strategies and to rejuvenate the Programme. This literature gives a country scenario with special reference to West Bengal malaria problem and its control along with brief descriptions of the current drug and insecticide policies.

Introduction

Malaria is one of the major public health problems not only in West Bengal, but also in India. The history of control of malaria in India has seen tremendous success as well as failures. The disease, which has been responsible for considerable degree of morbidity and mortality during the pre-independence period continues its onslaught on the health and economy of the country during the early years of post-independence of India.

* Joint Director (Entomology), Regional Office for Health and Family Welfare, Govt. of India, 49/12B Hindusthan Park, Kolkata-700029

The tremendous success of National Malaria Control Programme (1953) with residual spray with DDT and the subsequent follow-up measures under the National Malaria Eradication Programme (1958) has helped the country to recover in economic fronts. Since 1974, several parts of India is under the grip of malaria.

Status of Malaria in India

Background

Malaria is a disease of great socio-economic importance. In past, this deadly disease has prevented from invasion into new areas. It can destroy whole national economy. For example, the great Mughal Army could not penetrate deep into Assam due to several reasons in which malaria is one. Sinton in 1935 estimated that economic loss due to malaria at the time of independence of India (1947) was about Rupees 7500 million per annum.

In 1947, it was estimated that 75 million people suffer from the disease every year. The mortality due to malaria was placed at 0.8 million per annum. The then Govt. of India implemented National Malaria Control Programme (NMCP) from 1953 which started large scale DDT spray till 1956 and brought down child and infant parasite rates by 79% and 62% respectively. The specticular success of NMCP led to launch into a National Malaria Eradication Programme (NMEP) since April, 1956. The success of NMEP was very much evident in 1967 when only 50,000 malaria cases without any death were noted in India. In 1962, after independent appraisals by International teams NMEP entered consolidation and maintenance phase.

During 1966, 50% areas of the country, from where malaria was practically eradicated and the vertical organisation of NMEP was withdrawn and public health services were made responsible for malaria free status. Thereafter, there was a gradual increase during the subsequent years and by 1976, the total number of cases recorded were 6.4 million. The programme was reviewed in depth and modified plan of operation was instructed in 1977 i.e. all malaria control activities were initiated from Primary Health Centre level. Laboratories were decentralised to PHC level. Large number of Drug distributing Centres (DDC) and fever treatment depots (FTD) opened in sub-centre and village level. Insecticidal spray during the transmission period in rural areas and introduction of fortnightly domicillary visit, blood smear collection and treatment system had led to significant reduction in malaria incidence to a level of 2 million cases per annum by 1984.

Between 1994 and 1996, there were malaria outbreaks in several areas of India. The programme strategy was again reviewed in 1995 by an Expert Committee, prioritising high risk areas for control epicdemics and use selective methods of vector control. It was felt by the experts that in this present set-up along with rapid changes in behaviour of parasite and vector, it is difficult to eradicate malaria. This change in concept, underlying malaria control, is least signified by the nomenclatural changes in the programme to control malaria in India, when in 1998 National Malaria Eradication Programme (NMEP) got changed to National Anti-Malaria Programme (NAMP).

Since long NAMP is not only responsible for malaria control but also responsible for prevention and control of Filaria, Kala-azar, Japanese Encephalitis and Dengue/DHF. Therefore, in order to keep better about the integrated scheme, since December, 2003 NAMP has again been renamed as "National Vector Borne Diseases Control Programme" (NVBDCP).

Present status

(1) Status of India

After implementation of MPO, the incidence of malaria in India is limited to 1.79 million (1986) to 3.04 (1996) per annum. The incidences of malaria in India since 1986 to 2002 are given in Table-1. The National Annual Blood Examination rate varies between 9.1 to 10.5 which is acceptible level. Although total malaria cases varies between 1.7 million to 3.04 million, but, from Table-1 it may be mentioned that *Plasmodium falciparum* infection along with death due to malaria shows a remarkable increasing trend. In 1987, only 0.62 million *P.falciparum* cases with 188 confirmed death due to malaria were noted in India, but in 1999 *P.falciparum* cases and death due to malaria increased to 1.14 million and 1048 respectively. This drew the attention of malariologist in India. During 1998, there was a decline in total malaria cases by 16.4% whereas *P. falciparum* cases has shown marginal increase by 2.26% as compared to 1997. Further, during 1999, there was a marginal increase in total cases by 2.79% whereas *P. falciparum* cases has shown substantial increase by 10.8% as compared to 1998. However, during 2002 total number of malaria cases showed below two million.

Table 1 : Epidemiological Situation of Malaria in India

Year	Blood Slide Examined (million)	Malaria cases (million)	P.falciparum (million)	ABER	SPR	Death
1976	55.98	6.47	0.75	9.73	11.55	59
1986	67.69	1.79	0.64	9.18	2.65	323
1987	72.53	1.66	0.62	9.63	2.29	188
1988	75.70	1.85	0.68	9.87	2.45	209
1989	72.07	2.05	0.76	9.37	2.84	268
1990	74.42	2.02	0.75	9.49	2.71	353
1991	75.16	2.12	0.92	9.30	2.82	421
1992	79.01	2.13	0.88	9.59	2.69	422
1993	77.94	2.21	0.85	9.35	2.83	354
1994	82.18	2.51	0.99	9.54	3.06	1122
1995	83.52	2.93	1.14	9.40	3.50	1151
1996	91.54	3.04	1.18	10.49	3.32	1010
1997	89.45	2.66	1.01	10.11	2.97	879
1998	NA	2.22	1.03	9.50	2.45	664
1999	NA	2.28	1.14	NA	NA	1048
2000	87.12	2.02	1.05	NA	2.32	931
2001	88.04	2.08	1.01	NA	2.25	1005
2002 (P)	NA	1.82	NA	NA	NA	902

* NA : Data not available.

* (P) : Provisional data as on 15.7.2003

Table-2 shows the State and Union Territory wise incidence pattern of malaria in India from 1998 to 2002. In the year 2002 Orissa State contributing highest i.e., 25.6% of malaria and more than 50% death due to malaria in comparison to India. The high malaria cases reporting States are Madhya Pradesh, Assam, Chhattisgarh, Gujarat, Karnataka, West Bengal, Jharkhand, Arunachal Pradesh etc.

Table 2: Reported Cases and Deaths Due to Malaria

	1998		1999		2000		2001		2002*	
State/U.T.	PC	D	PC	D	PC	D	PC	D	PC	D
Andh. Pr.	118800	12	129020	11	80557	6	57735	1	38053	0
Arun. Pra.	49554	2	58243	1	46165	0	56030	14	46431	0
Assam	94645	34	131048	111	84915	43	95142	122	89601	72
Bihar	114958	34	131898	131	9509	2	4108	0	3683	2
Chattisga.					359155	63	29066	32	245365	3
Goa	25975	19	15380	17	9164	11	12331	12	16818	15
Gujrat	106825	3	64130	7	36712	2	81347	19	80983	9
Haryana	12115	0	2604	0	1050	0	1202	0	936	0
HP	1433	0	700	0	491	0	349	0	176	0
J & K	5451	0	3574	0	3045	0	912	0	477	0
Jharkhand					133453	16	130784	21	126589	31
Karnataka	118712	3	97274	11	109118	14	197625	21	132584	35
Kerala	7439	7	5141	7	2940	9	2289	9	2985	8
MP	475098	26	527510	50	194689	93	183118	81	108818	30
Maharashtra	165985	32	137712	46	81406	40	56043	50	45568	43
Manipur	1306	1	2662	8	1064	0	943	5	1268	9
Meghalaya	17618	2	14798	5	13699	11	20630	17	17918	36
Mizoram	10137	56	14437	73	9059	37	10929	43	7859	35
Nagaland	1989	0	4396	12	3443	0	4318	1	3945	0
Orissa	478056	349	483095	399	509497	467	454541	305	468046	420
Punjab	5316	0	1113	0	493	1	604	0	250	0
Rajasthan	76438	0	53154	0	35973	10	129233	36	68627	11
Sikkim	15	0	14	0	16	0	31	0	53	0
Tamil Nadu	63915	2	56366	2	43053	1	31551	0	27337	0
Tripura	12595	5	14408	11	12245	6	18502	9	13322	5
Uttaranchal					2008	0	1196	0	1675	0
UP	112291	0	99362	0	96971	0	94524	15	90188	0
West Bengal	132088	77	227480	144	145322	103	145053	191	181272	139
A N Islands	1247	0	937	2	1002	1	925	1	865	1
Chandigarh	1675	0	456	0	256	0	298	0	157	0
D & N Haveli	6225	0	3303	0	2415	0	848	0	493	0
Daman & Diu	625	0	352	0	132	0	87	0	173	0
Delhi	4050	0	3996	0	2631	0	1484	0	694	0
Lakshdweep	4	0	1	0	5	0	0	0	8	0
Pondicherry	168	0	149	0	137	0	106	0	103	0
All India Total	2222748	664	2284713	1048	2031790	932	2085484	1005	1823320	902

*** Provisional (15.7.2003)**
PC = Positive Cases / D = Deaths

(2) *Malaria Status of West Bengal*

Geographically West Bengal occupies 2.7% of the landmass in compared to India. In 2002, West Bengal contributed 10.6% total malaria cases (total cases 1,94,421) in comparison to India (total cases 18,23,320). In the same year, West Bengal contributed 16.8% death due to malaria in compared to 902 death due to malaria in India. The epidemiological situation of malaria in West Bengal since 1990 to 2002 is shown in Table-3.

Table 3: Year wise Epidemiological Data on Malaria in West Bengal

Year	Surveillance pop. (in 000)	B.S. Examined (in 000)	B.S. +ve	P. f. cases	Pf%	Death due to Malaria	ABER	SPR	SFR	API
1990		1610	27531	3892	14.1	4	3.0	1.7	0.24	
1991		1845	40452	7913	19.6	13	3.1	2.2	0.43	
1992		2475	49130	9170	18.7	43	4.3	1.9	0.37	
1993		2078	46138	8723	18.9	37	3.4	2.2	0.42	
1994		2535	74283	15399	20.7	52	4.1	2.9	0.61	
1995		2528	91014	17226	18.9	87	4.0	3.6	0.68	
1996	63694	2448	87686	14731	16.8	54	3.8	3.6	0.60	
1997	65915	2093	79881	11480	15.2	74	3.1	3.8	1.80	
1998	79391	2426	132088	25156	19.0	77	3.0	5.4	1.73	
1999	82090	2881	227480	72755	32.0	144	3.5	7.9	2.5	
2000	82380	2983	145322	32465	22.3	116	3.6	4.9	1.1	1.76
2001	82380	3367	145053	42566	29.3	205	4.1	4.3	1.2	1.76
2002	83970	3896	194421	60726	31.2	152	4.9	4.9	1.5	2.34

B.S. = Blood Slide

P.F. = P. falciparum

Annual Blood Examination Rate (ABER) in West Bengal is very poor (varies between 3.0 to 4.9) indicating poor surveillance mechanism in the State. In spite of poor ABER incidence of malaria along with *P. falciparum* cases showing steady increasing trend till 1999. Total incidence of malaria showed decreasing trend by 36.1% and 0.2% in 2000 and 2001 respectively in relation to its corresponding years 1999 and 2000.

Although Malaria is prevailing in all 17 districts of West Bengal but maximum transmission of malaria is going on in the sub-himalayan districts- Jalpaiguri and Coochbehar of North Eastern West Bengal, Purulia, Midnapore and Bankura of South Western part of West Bengal specially the blocks adjacent of Singhbhum of Jharkhand and Sundargarh of Orissa. Malaria in Kolkata Municipal Corporation is contributing 27.7% of total malaria cases, 11.8% *P. falciparum* infection and 27.6% death due to malaria in comparison to 2001 West Bengal data is a classical example of urban malaria problem in country.

In 2002, (as per Table-4 *on page 28*), district Jalpaiguri alone contributed 40.3% total cases, 57.4% *P. falciparum* infection and 27.6% total death due to malaria in comparison to West Bengal figure. A total of 130.42% increase in cases noted in 2002 in comparison to 2001 figure.

Vector and its control

Anopheles stephensi is the only vector of malaria in Kolkata Municipal Corporation area. The vector breeds in numerous fresh water collections in domestic and peridomestic areas. The vector has already developed resistant to DDT, BHC and malathion.

At present anti vector measures by K.M.C. includes application of larvaecides like Baytex, Abate and Biocides in water along with irregular thermal fogging with pyrethrum in high affected areas. Mass I.E.C. compaign is also done along with Chaemotherapy through 42 malaria clinics and hospitals.

In the districts of Purulia, Midnapore and Bankura malaria is mainly prevalent in tribal areas. Where *A.culicifacies* and *A. fluviatilis* is the main vector. *A.culicifacies* transmits malaria in monsoon and post monsoon season, whereas *A.fluvatilis* transmits malaria in h illy areas in winter months. Two rounds DDT spraying is being done to control these species. *A. culicifacies* is noted as highly resistant to DDT, *A.fluviatilis* the other species, however, has been found to be susceptible to DDT.

In the districts like Jalpaiguri and Coochbehar multiple vectors playing roles in transmission of malaria. Near the forest areas, *A.dirus* is the primary vector. The other vectors are *A.fluviatilis* in the foot hills. *A. minimus* near tea gardens areas. *A.annularies* also acting as secondary vector. Two rounds DDT is being done to control malaria in these district. Mass IEC campaign for people co-operation and source reduction along with early diagnosis and prompt treatment is a primary component for malaria control in West Bengal.

Table 4: Selective District Wise Epidemiological Situation of Malaria in West Bengal

District	Year	No.+ve for malaria	PF%	Death (con-firmed)	ABER	SPR	SFR	Disease trend
	1999	32565	35.16	42	6.83	14.51	5.10	
Jalpaiguri	2000	20522	31.88	16	6.53	9.34	2.97	-36.98%
	2001	34000	46.09	38	9.38	10.71	4.96	+65.675%
	2002	78346	44.45	42	12.40	18.56	8.2	+130.42%
	1999	4375	18.86	12	4.09	4.27	0.80	
Coochbehar	2000	3870	9.27	02	5.84	2.58	0.24	-11.54%
	2001	5213	15.49	15	6.88	2.95	0.45	+34.70%
	2002	5624	19.44	14	7.62	2.88	0.5	+7.92%
	1999	15125	31.87	19	9.44	7.29	2.32	
Purulia	2000	25126	27.15	14	9.97	9.68	2.63	+66.12%
	2001	22565	29.0	19	9.58	9.05	2.63	-10.19%
	2002	16772	58.8	04	11.30	5.70	3.3	-25.67%
	1999	3851	24.92	02	4.24	0.94	0.23	
Midnapore	2000	2447	21.41	01	4.19	0.60	0.13	-36.458%
	2001	3760	22.81	01	4.15	0.95	0.21	+53.658%
	2002*	5002	32.10	01	2.96	1.71	0.5	+33.03%
	1999	2554	30.19	00	6.87	1.17	0.35	
Bankura	2000	3917	42.37	03	8.04	1.58	0.67	+53.37%
	2001	2398	6.38	06	8.54	0.91	0.05	-38.78%
	2002	1188	35.40	10	9.35	0.40	0.1	-50.45%
	1999	149691	32.61	68	9.66	32.8	10.67	
Kolkata	2000	84438	19.05	55	7.17	24.8	4.72	-43.59%
(K.M.C.)	2001	71807	23.63	83	7.47	20.3	4.8	-14.959%
	2002	53951	13.31	42	4.85	24.2	3.2	-24.86%
	1999	227480	32.0	144	3.50	7.9	2.50	
W. Bengal	2000	145322	22.3	116	3.60	4.9	1.08	-36.12%
	2001	145053	29.3	205	4.10	4.3	1.26	-0.185%
	2002	194421	31.23	152	4.96	4.9	1.5	+34.03%

* *Data included both for East and West Midnapore Districts.*

Malaria control strategies

The ecosystem of our country has been constantly changıng due to various developmental activities, leading to the changing epidemiological pattern of malaria. Increased *P.falciparum* cases and mortality due to malaria, specially in urban and tribal areas of India causing a great concerned to public health worker. Honourable Prime Minister of India on 5th December, 1994 reviewed the programme and advised for a new direction to the programme Union Ministry of Health and Family Welfare, appointed an expert committee in December, 1994. The committee submitted its report on 27th January, 1995, known as Malaria Action Programme (MAP'95)

The objectives are:

1. Effective control of malaria to bring reduction in malaria morbidity.
2. Prevention of death due to malaria.
3. Consolidation of gains achieved so far.

Apart from the above objectives capacity building of various levels of personnel has also been taken up in big way new under the programme. The involvement of community by IEC activities and by mass mobilisation campaigns during the anti-malaria month in June of every year is now a major plank of control strategy. These temporal changes in concepts, underlying malaria control are best signified by the nomenclatural changes, in the programme to control malaria in India from National Malaria Eradication Programme to National Anti Malaria Programme, which in December, 2002 is renamed as National Vector Borne Diseases Programme.

To achieve these objectives following strategies recommended to intensify malaria control activities throughout the countries with focus on "High Risk Areas" through an integrated malaria control stategies which has the following components:

1. Early case detection and prompt treatment (EDPT).
2. Selective vector control.
3. Promotion of personal protection method.
4. Early detection and containment of epidemics.
5. Information, education and communication (IEC) towards personal prevention and community participation.
6. Institutional and management capacity building, trend manpower development and efficient management and information system (MIS).

Identificaiton of "High Risk" areas

In order to identify worst affected "High risk" malarious areas the Expert Committee has laid down the following criteria in rural areas.

a. Record of indegenous death due to malaria.

b. Doubling of slide positivity rate (SPR) during last three years provided the SPR in second on third year reaches 4% or more.

c. Where SPR does not show the doubling trend as above but the average SPR of the last three years is 5% or more.

d. *P falciparum* proportion is 30% or more provided the SPR is 3% or more.

e. An area having a focus of Chloroquine resistant *P. falciparum* cases.

f. Tropical aggregation of labour in Project areas, new settlements on tourist areas.

Case detection and management of malaria cases

Early diagnosis and prompt treatment is most important activity at the periphery for preventing malaria mortality. Apart from existing case detection and treatment centres, Govt. of India emphasised on opening more Drug Distributing Centres (DDC) and Fever Treatment Depots (FTD) in village level and more Malaria clinics in Urban areas.

The National Anti Malaria Drug Policy was first drafted in 1982 by National Expert Team to combat the increasing level of resistance to chloroquine detected in *P.falciparum* and prevent death due to malaria.

Presently the following anti-malarials are available:

1. Schizonticidal drugs for clinical and parasitological cure are chloroquine, Amodiaquine, Quinine, Quinidine, Pyremethamine, Trimethoprim, Proguanil, Sulfonamides in combination with Pyremethamine, Mefloquine, Halofantrine, Artemisinine.

2. Gametocidal and anti-relapse drug is primaquine, 8-aminoquinolines group.

Among these drugs Chloroquine is considered as the drug of choice because it has a rapid action on schizonts, lease toxic with very few adverse effect.

Expert Committee recommended that,

a. The first line of treatment is chloroquine and the second line is sulfaleme/sulfadoxine pyremethamine combination. In case of resistant to these two drugs and in severe and complicated malaria quinine will be used.

b. All suspected malaria cases should be presumptively administered 25 mg/kg. bd. wt. of chloroquine base over 3 days with a single dose of Primaquine 0.75 mg./kg. This drug regime is to be followed up to the sub centre level throughout the country limited to the high risk areas. In the low risk areas and DDC and FIDs in all areas would continue to provide presumptive treatment with 10 mg/kg.bd., wt. chloroquine single dose.

c. The dose of Primaquine for *P.vivax* cases is 0.25mg./kg. daily for 5 days to prevent relapse and for *P. falciparum* 0.75mg./kg. single dose for gametocidal action. Where presumptive treatment with primaquine has been given in sensitive areas as a second dose with it will not be required.

d. Amodiaquine has not advantage over chloroquine resistant areas and considering the toxicity associated with it, amodiaquine may be withdrawn from the programme.

Vector control

To generate detail data on vector bionomics and to note susceptibility status of vectors to insecticides from PHC level 72 entomological zones established under Modified Plan of Operation of which only 32 zones are functioning with complete staff strength. In West Bengal there are three zones i.e. Jalpaiguri, Burdwan and Kolkata. The posts of Assistant Entomologist in all the three zones are vacant and acute shortage of infrastructural facilities.

Keeping in view the difficulties encountered by the zonal entomological teams, supports have been made by NAMP through World Bank supported Enhanced Malaria Control Project (EMCP) in the States of Andhra Pradesh, Bihar, Gujrat, Madhya Pradesh, Maharashtra, Orissa and Rajasthan.

Vector control policy

Vector control policy is distinctly divided by vector control in urban areas and vector control in rural areas.

Presently the spray operations with different insecticides are being carried out in all areas with Annual Parasite Index (API) of 2 or more. The priority of spray is being given to "High Risk Areas" all over the country. In high risk areas the epidemilogical data of proceeding three years are considered for selecting the population protected.

Although several malaria vectors, specially *A. culicifacies* found resistant to DDT, is should be the insecticide of choice for mayn reasons.

The other insecticide BHC has been used extensively in the public health for disease control programmes and agriculture. The vectors developed resistant to it. Govt. of India withdraw BHC from public health since 1997.

It has been decided by Expert Committee that if a vector develop resistant to DDT, Malathion would be the alternative insecticide. If vectors develop double resistant to DDT and malathion, then third alternative insecticide to be sprayed is synthetic pyrethroids (i.e. Deltamethrin, Cyfluthrin, Lambdacyhalothrin etc).

Recently experts of Government of India given more importance to use of insecticides (Synthetic pyrethroid) impregnated bed-nets in night in order to give more protection and to present death. The control strategies are,

Vector control in urban areas

a. Residual spray is not advocated for control of adult mosquitoes due to high refusal rate and environment pollution problem.

b. Pyrethrum space spray is not advocated, but in emergency it can be done to control epidemic situation specially in *P. falciparum* area.

c. Water management should be done by providing appropriate water supply and disposal.

d. Improvement of storm water drainage.

e. Source reduction of peridomestic water bodies.

f. Implementation of civic by laws.

g. Anti larval measures with larvaecides (Baytex, temophos etc.)/ Biocides or application of larvaevorous fishes like Gambusia, Poicela etc.

h. Promotion of use of bed-nets, specially insecticide treated nets during sleeping.

Vector control in rural areas

a. Water management by intersectorial co-ordination.

b. Pyrethrum space spray for immediate control of epidemic by *P.falciparum* infection.

c. In difficult tribal dominated malarious areas, if the people have the habit of sleeping outdoor they should be provided with synthetic pyrethroid treated bed nets.

d. DDT is still the insecticide of choice, where vectors are susceptible to DDT. If the vector resistant to DDT (Entomological and Epidemiological findings) malathion should be sprayed. Where vector/s are multiple resistant to DDT, malathion synthetic pyrethroid may be sprayed indoor (not cattlesheds to be sprayed) residual spray.

The successful implementation of any programme is often attributed to community involvement and the inter-sectoral co-ordination with different sectors of economy. Keeping this in view, the Directorate of NAMP initiated the concept of observation of Antimalaria month in June every year. The main objectives of Anti malaria month in all over the country are (1) to create awareness among the community (2) to establish community involvement in prevention of malaria and (3) to propogate the theme "Malaria Control : Everyone's Concern".

In the meantime, all State Governments were initiated to form State level Task Force along with formation of District and Block level co-ordination committees for control of malaria with an objective to prepare micro level plan of action and to identify high and low risk subcentres.

Govt. of India has already started country-wise training programmes for different level of Government personnels in order to build up their capacity for successfully control of malaria.

References

- Annon (1986) "Malaria and its control in India"-Vol. I. *Directorate of National Malaria Eradication Programme, Directorate General of Health Services, Government of India.* 1-346.
- Annon (1995) "Operational manual for malaria action programme, Govt. of India National Malaria Eradiction Programme, Ministry of Health and F.W., 22, Sham Nath Marg, Delhi-110054. 1-180.
- Mukhopadhyay A.K., Karmaker P.K., Hati A.K. and Dey P. (1997) "Recent epidemiological status of malaria in Calcutta Municipal Corporation areas, West Bengal, *India J. Mal.* **34** 186-196.
- Mukhopadhyay A.K., Hati A.K., Dey P. (2000) "Malariogenic situations amounting to premonition in areas of Ajodhya Hills of District Purulia, West Bengal". *J. Common. Dis.* **32** (3) 231-233.
- Pattanayak, S., Sharma V.P., Kalra N.L., Orlov, V.S., Sharma R.S. (1994) "Malaria Paradims in India and Control Strategy" *India J. Mal* 31 (**4**). 141-170.

- Sharma R.S., Sharma G.K., Dhillon G.P.S. (1996) "Epidemiology and control of malria in India"- *Ministry of Health and Family Welfare, Dte. of National Malaria Programme.* 1-751.
- Shivlal, Dhillon G.P.S., Sonal G.S., Rama Rao, Sita B. (1998) "Country Scenario malaria and its control in India. March, 1998. *National Malaria Eradication Programme (EMCP), Dte. General of Health Services, 22, Sham Nath Marg, Delhi-110054,* pp. 1-98.
- Sinton J.A. (1935) what malaria costs India nationally, socially and economically, *Rec. Mal. Surv. Ind.,* 5 **(3)** : 224-264.

Chapter - 3

Development of Micro Area Malaria Control Strategy : A Case study in Kolkata

** Jayanta Basu*

Abstract

Malaria has come back with increased vengenence after a period of apparent subsidence during 1960s. In view of the changing situation, the strategy of malaria control has been suitably modified throughout the world under the umbrella of World Health Organisation (WHO). The situation has further complicated due to the fact that malaria has become increasingly urbane in nature. Kolkata is no exception, contributing about 50% of the overall malaria cases in the state. With this background the author has been carrying out a study on behalf of a NGO for over last five years in collaboration with number of govt. & non govt. agencies. The findings have led to the development of a malaria control model named "MICRO AREA MALARIA CONTROL STRATEGY" (MAMCS) to be implemented with the support of target community. The model has been applied in the Pyarabagan Slum area of south Kolkata during 1999-2000 and consequently MAMCS for the area has been developed.

Introduction

Malaria, one of the deadliest public health hazard ever to affect mankind, has come back with increased vengenence after a period of apparent subsidence during 1960s. Within a period of few years, the euphoria over mosquito eradication through application of DDT and efficacy of wonder drug chloroquinine has evaporated and malaria has come back stronger than ever. Mosquitoes have been reported to be building up resistance against DDT and so does the *Plasmodium* parasites against chloroquinine drug. In view

* Environment Governed Intergrated Organisation, 26/1, Ramesh Mitra Road, G. Floor, Kolkata-700 025.

of the changing situation, the strategy of malaria control has been modified throughout the world under the umbrella of World Health Organisation (WHO). The mosquito eradication programme has given way to more pragmatic mosquito control programme and antimalarial drug regime has been suitably modifed. India is no exception. Over the last 30 years, the malaria situation has undergone qualitative as well as quantitative changes in the country. In addition to increasingly higher SPR (Slide Positivity Rate), the Pv: Pf index has gone up in favour of latter. Moreover, malaria has gradually become more and more urbane in nature. Kolkata is no exception. It is an established fact that now more than 50% malaria cases throughout West Bengal actually occur within Kolkata Municipal Corporation (KMC) area. The unplanned urbanisation coupled with less than adequate health delivary system and abundance of anophiline mosquito vectors are believed to be the chief causes behind this phenomenon.

A study carried out by the author on behalf of Environment Governed Integreted Organisation (EnGIO) in collaboration and/or support of different govt. and non govt. organisations including Kolkata municipal corporation; Kolkata and State Police; WWF Nature India; Malaria Directorate, Govt. of West Bengal and others for over last four years revealed that incidence of malaria is actually related to number of factors' like status of awareness level; socio-economic condition; *per capita* night time space etc. The study, being carried out in different reportedly malaria-prone areas of KMC, has yielded interesting findings and observation which, in brief, are as follows :

- Areawise variability of malarial incidence pattern (even within very small geographical areas).
- General lack of awareness regarding malaria.
- Lack of awareness seems to be directly related to high malaria incidence pattern.
- High night time density per room is a contributing factor against under usage of mosquito nets and thus higher malaria rate.
- Dominance of *Plasmodium falciparum* (Pf) over *Plasmodium vivax (Pv)* during certain period of the year.

It has been found that due to the heterogenous character of city, most of the mentioned parameters show localised variation. In view of these findings, it seems that no blanket malaria control strategy will work in the city and a 'MICRO AREA MALARIA

CONTROL STRATEGY' (MAMCS) needs to be developed keeping in mind the status of local parameters. Involvement of all stake holders including the exposed community, at both strategy formulation and implementation stages, is an absolute necessity for successful adoption and implementation of the same.

With this background, the present 3½ months study has been undertaken in ward no. 69 and 72 with Pyarabagan Slum as the focal point for development of MAMCS.

Pyarabagan slum and around : A case study of *MAMCS*

The particular area has been chosen as study area for pilot programme due to two reasons, the area being highly malariogenic with very low awareness level as found out on the basis of previous studies. As a matter of fact the Pyarabagan slum happens to be one of the biggest slum areas of the city holding more than five thousand people. Moreover, the civic conditions of the slum are quiet poor though Kolkata Municipal Corporation has recently started some works relating to drainage and other civic facilities under an Asian Development Bank (ADB) supported project named 'Kolkata Environment Improvement Project' (KEIP).

The ongoing malaria control project has been a joint initiative of two non-profit organisations namely 'South Asian Foundation for Human Initiatives' (SAFHI) and 'Environment Governed Integrated Organisation' (EnGIO), later providing the technical support. The major objective of the project was two fold:

(a) To spread awareness regarding malaria within target population.

(b) To develop MAMCS for the project area with the help of data generated from the study.

Methodology

The study has been carried out in ward no. 69 & 72 of KMC with Pyarabagan slum area as its focal point. The area has been selected on the basis of the studies carried out in the area over the last 3 years, which justified a comprehensive study regarding malarial dynamics in said zone.

The 3 & 1/2 months study initiated at 15 November, 1999 had in all 2100 respondent households, 1600 included in the main sutdy and 500 in awareness evaluation study. The study has been conducted by one project supervisor and three field workers through a pre-structured and pre-tested questionnaire. The entire sample has been broadly divided into slum and non slum areas.

2/3 of the respondents were from the focal area i.e. slum whereas rest 1/3 were from the peripheral zone. The respondents have been selected randomly by the field workers based on unbiased zone mapping. The broad activities are as follows:

Questionnaire survey and awareness generation

The phase-I field activity included questionnaire survey and awareness generation regarding malaria with distribution of the Information, Education and Communication (IEC) materials. The Phase-II field activity i.e. evaluation of awareness generation has been recorded in the last 15 days of the project, from the sample which has already been exposed to Phase-I.

The Phase I questionnaire included queries about age, sex, educational status, employment, socio-economic status, malarial history in family, mode of treatment etc.

The phase-II questionnaire included the queries regarding source of malaria, usage/non-usage of mosquito nets and mosquito repellants, storage of water, disease response pattern etc.

Detection of malaria

Collection of blood samples within target population had been carried out throughout the project tenure from the fixed point at project office and also directly from households and temporary sample collection points within project area. Both thick and thin blood smears were taken for each patient, subsequently tested by a support organisation, Mediprobe Pathology and Research Centre. Giemsa stain has been used to stain the slide. After detailed observation of both the thick and thin smears, reports have been prepared and sent to the project office in the same evening, so that they can be collected by the affected persons facilitating early treatment, if required.

Vector study

Certain species of anophiline mosquito are the vectors for innoculation and transmission of malaria. Worldwide one of the acceptable mode of malaria control is to control the vectors. As controlling the adult mosquito population has universally accepted as quiet difficult hence the larvae control is widely adopted. As a matter of fact the anophiline larval dynamics in a particular area is a pointer vis-a-vis the area's vulnerability to the malarial incidence. In the current study lot of emphasis had been put to study the larval dynamics of the study area.

Actually three modes of larvae detection methods have been simultaneously applied in the study. Firstly, a house specific larvae detection survey along with the questionnaire survey had been undertaken, with experienced field workers assigned for the job. Secondly, a possible water accumulation points including containers of various sizes and shapes, tanks etc. were studied for the purpose. Parallely, a control experiment was set up within project area to study the larval dynamics by regularly monitoring the larvae quantitatively and qualitatively from ten clear water filled containers kept in certain points within the same.

Thirdly, a region vulnerability study with respect to larvae breeding and propagation was undertaken through a qualititative assessment of the area through identifying the possible and/or potential source points for large scale mosquito breeding.

The MAMCS for the target population has been prepared on the basis of the study findings and the same has been finalised with input from the community representatives. The participation and active involvement of all stake holders including target community in MAMCS development have been ensured by regular interactions through LMRT (Local Malaria Round Table) and FGD (Focussed Group Discussion)

Results and Interpretation

The results are shown in tabular forms

Profile of malaria detection

Table 1 : Malaria Detection Dynamics within Study Area

Period	BSE	SPR	MAL.POS.	Pv	Pf	PV:Pf	GAMETOCYTE
Nov, '99	79	60%	50	29	21	3:2	2
Dec, '99	223	25%	56	9	47	1:5	8
Jan, 2000	356	15%	53	13	40	1:3	3
Feb, 2000	347	20%	69	56	13	4:1	2
Nov, '99 to Feb, 2000	**1005**	**23%**	**228**	**107**	**121**	**1:1.1**	**15**

BSE : Blood Sample Examined; SPR : Slide Positivity Rate

Interpretation of the results

Out of the total BSE of 1005 spread over 3 and 1/2 months (Mid November, 1999 to February end, 2000), the overall SPR (Slide Positivity Rate) has been found to be 23% with Pv : Pf about 1: 1.1.

However, this statistics showed wide ranging departure from month to month. For example the SPR is as high as 60% in November 1999 and as low as 15% in January 2000.

The Pv : Pf ratio also deviated significantly being about 1:5 in December 1999 (in favour of Pf), while it is 4:1 in February, 2000 (in favour of Pv). All these datas indicate the very fluid state of malarial dynamics within study area which may be related to the seasonal changes. Another interesting point to note is that about 15 cases out of total 228 positives were found to carry gametocytes stages meaning about 6.5% of the positive cases detected, fall within career category and this individuals will be largely responsible for restarting the cycle allover again if not properly treated at the earliest.

Table-2: Household Malarial Dynamics Within Sampled Population

Area	Sample Size	HouseHold Positive	HouseHold Negative	Hospital-isation	Mortality
Focal	1044	1012	32	188	8
	100	97	3	-	-
Peripheral	556	517	39	9	1
	100	93	7	-	-
Overall	1600	1529	71	197	9
	100	95.5	4.5	-	-

Table-3: Malarial Awareness Profile Within Study Population

Area	Sample Size	Fully Aware	Partly Aware	Non Aware	Mosquito Net Use Pattern		Source Knowledge	
					User	Non User	Have	Don't Have
Focal	1044	58	252	734	308	736	470	574
	100	5.5	24.1	70.4	29.5	70.5	45	55
Peripheral	556	30	193	333	223	333	445	111
	100	5.4	34.7	59.9	40.1	59.9	80	20
Overall	1600	88	445	1067	531	1069	915	685
	100	5.5	27.8	66.7	33.2	66.8	57	43

Table-4: Sleeping Profile of Study Population

Area	Sample Size	Indoor Sleeping Habit	Outdoor Sleeping Habit (Occasional+Always)
Focal	1044	1033	11
	100	99	1
Peripheral	556	556	-
	100	100	-
Overall	1600	1589	11
	100	99.3	0.7

Table-5: Treatment Seeking Behaviour of Study Population Alongwith Symptom Classification

Area	Sample size	Treatment Seeking Behaviour		Symptoms				Health facility use		
		Seek	Non-Seek	F+H	F+H +V	F+V	Ors	Govt.	Pvt./ Qk	Both
Focal	1044	1033	11	742	44	182	76	385	558	90
	100	99	1	71.3	4.3	17.5	6.9	37.2	54	8.8
Peripheral	556	555	1	275	237	9	35	101	444	10
	100	99.99	0.01	49.5	42.8	1.5	6.15	18.1	80	1.9
Overall	1600	1588	12	101	281	191	111	486	1002	100
	100	99.3	0.7	63.6	17.5	11.9	7	30.6	63	6.4

Table-6: Study of Night time Room Density Within Sample Population

Area	Sample Size (Room)	1-3 Per Room	4-5 Per Room	6 & above Per Room
Focal	1044	43	417	584
	100	4	40	56
Peripheral	556	305	223	28
	100	55	42	3
Overall	1600	348	640	612
	100	21.7	40	38.3

Findings

Phase -I Detailed Questionnaire Survey

Table-1: Demographic Profile of Respondent Population

Area	Sample Size	Resp. Sex		Resp. Age	M.Tongue			Education			Employment		Socio.Eco.			Family Size		
		M	F		Ben	Hin	Ors	No.	SFDr.	SF& Ab.	Emp.	Un.	1000 & less pm	1000 to 3000 pm	3000 & ab pm	1 to 4	5 to 7	8 & ab
Focal	1044	300	744	AllAd.	792	208	44	506	434	104	487	557	132	707	205	412	477	155
	100	28.7	71.3	100 Ad.	75.9	19.9	4.2	48.4	41.7	9.9	46.6	53.4	12.6	67.8	19.6	39.5	45.6	4.9
Perip-	556	332	224	All Ad.	426	120	10	156	201	199	278	278	26	388	142	248	251	57
heral	100	59.6	40.4	100Ad.	76.7	21.7	1.6	28.2	36.1	35.7	50	50	4.8	69.7	25.5	44.7	44.9	10.4
Over-	1600	632	968	All Ad.	1218	328	54	662	635	303	765	835	158	1095	347	660	728	212
all	100	39.5	60.5	100Ad.	76.2	20.5	3.3	41.4	39.7	18.9	47.8	52.2	9.9	68.4	21.7	41.2	45.5	13.3

Phase -II

Evaluation Survey

Table-7: Result of Evaluation Survey Within Study Population

Sample Size	Disease Source Knowledge		Source of Awareness		Mosquito Net Usage		
	Present	Absent	Newspaper TV/Project	Others/	Regular	Irregular	Non
550	500	50	522	28	242	5	303
100	91	9	95	3	44.1	0.9	55

Sample Size	Cause of Non Mosquito Net use		Repelent Use		Cause of Non Repelent use		
	Space Shortage	Don't Required	User	Non User	Suffocation	High Cost	Both
550	272	31	523	27	7	8	12
100	90	10	95	5	25.9	29.6	44.5

Sample Size	Response to Fever		Completion of Dose	
	Physicians	others	Yes	No
550	539	11	544	6
100	98	2	99	1

Interpretation of the results

The questionnaire based study clearly shows certain salient features of study population, which are as follows:

a. Very poor educational and socio-economic status of study population especially the population of focal area, with significantly high average family size.

b. Very high malaria incidence rate within both focal and peripheral zone population.

c. Very poor awareness level regarding malaria with significant low mosquito net users and low rate of mosquito source knowledge.

d. Primarily indoor sleeping habit.

e. More dependence on private health delivery system.

f. Night time density per room is quite high mainly in focal area maximising the probability of mosquito bite as mosquito nets cannot be used due to shortage of space.

From the above findings and/or observations it seems that the increase of awareness status in association with strengthening and standardization of malarial treatment and restructuring of sleeping pattern (if possible) may help to reduce the malaria menace.

Larvae Detection and Vulnerability Assessment

Table-1: Household Larvae Detection Profile

Area	H.H.S	N.Com-pl.	Com-pl.	Larve found	Period Nov.	Dec.	Jan.	Feb.	Cul+	Ano
Focal	1044	110	934	15	5	0	0	10	15	0
		10.54%	89.46%	1.61%	33%	-	-	67%	100	-
Peripheral	556	270	296	12	0	0	0	12	8	4
		48.56%	51.44%	4.44%	-	-	-	100%	67%	33%
Overall	1600	370	1230	27	5	0	0	22	23	4
		23.12%	76.88%	2.2%	18.5%	-	-	81.5%	85.2%	14.8%

Table-2: Study of Breeding Points

Month	Control Breeding Points									
	1	2	3	4	5	6	7	8	9	10
Nov	P*a	A	A	A	P*c	A	A	A	A	A
Dec	A	A	A	A	A	A	A	A	A	A
Jan	A	A	A	A	A	A	A	A	P*c	A
Feb	P**a	A	A	P*c	P*c	A	A	A	P*c	P**c

Control Breeding Points:*

1. B. Ed. College
2. Project Office
3. Padmapukur
4. Motor Vehicles
5. Pearabagan 1 (Wall-side)
6. Pearabagan 2 (Central Part)
7. Telephone Exchange
8. Taxi Union Office
9. Townshed Road
10. Ramesh Mitra Road

P - Present
A - Absent
* - Few
** - Moderate
a - Anopheles Larvae
c - Culicine Larvae

* *All the control breeding points are located within an approxiamate area of 4 km^2.*

Table-3 Study of Region Vulnerability With Respect to Potential Larvae Breeding Points

Vulnerable points	Cause of Vulnerability with respect to larvae breeding
* Motor Vechicles Compound	Multiple accommodation points including tyres, car parts, scrap materials/ undisturbed environment
* Ballygunge Police Station Compound	Do
* Beltala Garage	Do
* The peripheral and other parts of Pearabagan Slum. (Mainly disposal points)	Varieties of accommodation points like coconut shell, leftover containers etc./ moderately undisturbed environment
* David Hare College Compound	Fountain, fixed water source, construction work / undisturbed environment
* Ballygunge Government High School Compound	Tank, virtually stagnant sewerage
* Military Campus	During monsoon water may remain accmulated undisturbed for a prolonged period over a large area
* Ladies Park	Do
* 21, Chakraberia Road	Fountain
* Vats (behind Ladies Park)	Multiple sources like coconut shell, earthenwares/undisturbed environment
* Telephone exchange compound	Multiple sources remain scattered throughout especially in the back portion/ undisturbed environment
* Garages (at Ramesh Mitra Road)	Tyres, different containers remains scattered
* Garage (slum - General)	Do
* Slum at Gour Ghosh Road	Tank, virtually closed sewerage, broken earthenware, tyres etc.

* Indra Roy Road	Ongoing construction work
* Slum at Madhab Lane	Earthenware, tank etc.
* St. Lawrence Campus	Multiple breeding sources in undisturbed environment
* Central Govt. Employee quarters (opposite St. Lawrence)	Do
* Ballygunge Science College Compound	Do
* Building complexes like Saptapami, Nabakailash and others	Do

Interpretation of the results

Three parellel studies carried out for detection of actual and/or potential breeding sources of mosquito larvae wrt occurrence and spread of malaria have yielded very important findings which can be corelated. The salient features of the findings are as follows:

a) From the microlevel survey it has been found that the households of the focal zone i.e. slum area, are less vulnerable to that of the households in peripheral zone (multistoried buildings & others) vis-a-vis acting as the breeding sources of the anophiline mosquitoes, responsible for malaria.

b) Due to climatic and other conditions mosquito larvae, in general, are scarecely found from November onwards. However larvae are again found from February onwards though culicine larvae are much more predominant in occurrance.

c) It seems that the public places are more vulnerable to private places with respect to acting as breeding sources of mosquitoes as they remain largely unattended and uncared for. The region vulnerability study shows that the public places like motor vehicles, Police station etc. along with large multistoried buildings of the area may act as the reservior of vectors.

Keeping in mind the above features it seems that a very agressive larvae control program should be undertaken mainly February onwards giving emphasis to the control in the households in peripheral zone and public places of the area as indicated. Community participation is very important in this aspect as it is virtually impossible for Govt. machinary to regularly check the public places for larvae. Small local community group can undertake the responsibility after being properly briefed and trained about the same.

Conclusion and strategy formulation

The MAMCS (MICROAREA MALARIA CONTROL STRATEGY) for the study area (ward no. 69 & 72 with Pyarabagan slum as the focal point and rest as peripheral zone) has been developed broadly through two exercises,

a) Generation of relevant primary and collection of secondary data within study zone;

b) Close interactions and exchange of information/ideas with all stake-holders to develop the strategy mainly on the basis of findings generated from the study.

While the part (a) has been elaborately discussed before, the part (b) has been undertaken mainly through two methods--

* Build up of LOCAL MALARIA ROUND TABLE (LMRT) & regular interactions with LMRT members and
* FOCUSSED GROUP DISCUSSION (FGD) with local community.

LMRT excercises

- The LMRT has been consisted of local community representatives; local doctors; local administration (inclusive of Kolkata Police and KMC) representatives and subject experts.
- Opinions/ Suggestions from Experts of Zoological Survey of india (ZSI); Kolkata Municipal Corporation (KMC); Malaria Directorate, Govt. of West Bengal; Dept. of Health, Govt. of West Bengal; Dept. of Environment, Govt. of West Bengal; Environment Cell, KMDA; Dept. of Environmental Sciences, Calcutta University; Entomologists; Protozoologists and Medical Biologists from eminent Institutions and other relevant sectors have been regularly sought and minor project protocol modifications have been undertaken, as and when required on the basis of the same.

The final aim of the project i.e. strategy formuation actually has been concluded with LMRT exercises with options of further LMRTs in near future. At the conclusion of the project, the study results and tentatively formulated strategy have been shared with subject experts in a seminar having representations form State Govt., School of Tropical Medicine; AIIPH&H; KMC; Directorate of Malaria; GOWB & others, which is latter finalised on the basis of the interactions.

FGD exercises

Several 'focussed group discussions' with local community members were held at different stages of the project and their version of the problem have been noted. It has been ensured that representations from the study zone including female representatives remain involved in the process. Some of the basic observations arising from these FGDs are as follows:

- People in general, are quite sceptical about the provided health facilities in general and malaria detection/treatment facility in particular.
- People seem to be having little faith in any programme related to malaria as they brought little remedies over the last few years.

  People are not at all amused by one off programme, which they feel, only give publicity to the organisers.
- The current project finds favour of the community due to its continual nature. They, in fact, want the program to continue, especially the free/highly discounted malaria detection and treatment (if possible) parts.
- People point towards the practical problems for not using mosquito nets etc.
- People want their problems to be communicated properly to relevant Govt. departments. In this context, they also mentioned the problems about bad sewerage system; lack of drinking water facility etc.
- A large chunk of community is ready to share part cost of any programme which will sincerely try to address their problems in general and malaria in particular.

Based on the findings/observations/suggestions as derived from LMRT and FGDs coupled with study findings, the following MAMCS has been developed for the study are (Pyarabagan Slum and adjoining areas).

Findings/Observations	Strategy
• Low education status; low socio economic conditions	Spread of informal education with emphasis on environmental health in general.
• Low awareness level	Aggressive micro and macro awareness generation.

• Compulsive non awareness with respect to mosquito net usage vis-a-vis low *per capita* night time space. Repellants used are not found to be very effective.	Cannot improve drastically/ have to take it in stride/ may be the use of mosquito repellents with better effectiveness and low indoor pollution is the answer, cost may be the inhibiting factor.
• Porous households allowing easy access of mosquitoes during night time/ doors broken or absent/ large gaps in wall.	Gaps can be filled up with fine mosquito nets to make the house hold as safe as possible during night time. Gaps in the wall may be filled with the help of recycled disposed plastics and similar material.
• Symptom preference	As 88% malaria patients have fever and vomiting, hence it may be considered as primary symptom for malaria (as corroborated by doctors) and given due importance/ presumptive treatment may be used under such conditions as advised by doctors.
• About 6.5% carriers and high malaria incidence.	EDPT (Early Detection, Prompt Treatment) should be strictly followed: Proper medicines with proper doses should be administered to patients.
• Inconsistency of treatment regime.	Local level treatment stadardisation exercises may be undertaken from a common platform with synergistic government and non government interactions.
• Decision makers mainly males.	Males have to be brought into awareness buildup activity along the female counterparts.
• Visit to native place	Cannot be controlled in general but a check method can be built up as part of a long term strategy.

• Multiple potential larvae generation sites around the area/ mainly in households in peripheral zones and public places around the area (as found in region vulnerability survey).	The identified 'region vulnerable points' may be strictly monitored throughout the year mainly monsoon and post monsoon/mobilisation of community should be given top priority in fixing this problem (may be in form of local malaria group), coupled with aggressive larvae kiling in identified points.
• Low compliance level in peripheral zone with respect to larvae detection.	Should be made mandatory by law.
• High hospitalisation rate for malaria.	To ensure early detection, representatives from the community may be trained for collecting blood and preparing smear (both thick and thin) facilitating early detection and thus early treatment.
• Evaluation result	Increased awareness regarding malarial source does not necessarily mitigate corresponding increase of mosquito net usage due to pragmatic compulsions/can be worked upon at micro level.
• High malaria incidence history; high proportion of Pf : Pv; mainly seeking help of private physicians.	Strengthening and networking of local health delivery system; standardisation of treatment and dosage through some one-platform activity (as mentioned before); perhaps giving provision of very low cost malaria detection centre and medicine round the year.
• Predominance of Pf parasites over Pv during Oct to Jan and vice-versa in other seasons.	Research should be under taken to specify the growth parameters of respective parasites by *in vitro* change of parameter/possible identification of specific proteins/enzymes/antibodies prevalent with respect to parasite types.

• Growing no. of carrier individuals; mainly Pf.	Research should be undertaken to analyse of blood immunoglobin profiles with high resolution techniques like 2D Gel electrophoresis to help in future antimalarial treatment. Institutions like Dept. of Envioronmental Sciences, CU, IICB (Indian Institute of Chemical Biology, ZSI (Zoological Survey of India) may be very useful for this kind of Research.

Concluding Remarks

MAMCS components as proposed for the study area should be implemented in a sequential and complimentary manner with a scope of regular monitoring and modification to maximize the probability of success of the strategy.

This Pyarabagan model can be replicated within malario-prone areas of the city to evolve area based malaria control strategies. The modern software technologies like Geographical Information System (GIS) can be used to make the collected informations more user friendly and thus qualitatively improving the decision making and implementation process regarding malaria control.

References

- Basu, J (2002), Application of *GIS* in malaria control : The Kolkata Model, *International Seminar on Information Technology in IIT* (Kharagpur).
- Basu, J (2002), Interim Report of the Project 'Development and Implementation of Malaria control Project in Calcutta and Howrah', submitted to *Dept. of Env., GOWB*.
- Basu, J (2001), Role of Built Environment in Malaria Control, International Seminar on Information Technology in *IIT (Kharagpur)*.
- Basu, J (2001), A Model of Malaria Control *vis-a-vis* Role of Community Awareness, Seminar on Malaria in Kolkata by *Calcutta Municipal Corporation and Environment Governed Intergrated Organisation*.
- Bretas Gustavo (2001) *Geographic Information Systems for the Study and Control of Malaria*.

- Bhattacharya, S., Saha, S. K. & Mukherjee, K. C. (1996), Epidemiological studies of malaria in relation to vectors on Calcutta (abs.) *XX International Conference of Entomology*, Italy.
- Chatterjee, K.D. (1952), *Human Parasites and Parasitic Diseases.*
- Das, S.K., Mitra, B., and Basu, J., A Report on the Changing Pattern of Malarial Incidence (both quantitative and qualitative) in Calcutta, *Seminar on Status of Environment in West Bengal* organised by Indian Geographical Foundation , Calcutta.
- Jeffrey G.M. (1966), Epidemiological significance of repeated infections with homologous and heterologous strains & species of *Plasmodium. Bull. WHO.*, **35** : 873-882.
- Philips, R. S. (1983), *Malaria,* Arnold Heinmann p. 58.
- Pramanik, M.K., Acharya, P.M.R., Ghosh, S. & Dutta Gupta, A.K. (1992), Mosquito fauna of West Bengal, India, 1. A Preliminary survey on the mosquito fauna of greater Calcutta & its suburbs. *Proc. of Zool. Soc.*, **45**. Suppl. A : 555-562.
- Reports of Calcutta Municipal Corporation, 1995-2002 (incoml.)
- Sadhu, M. (1998), Dynamics of Malaria in CMC area, *School of Tropical Medicine.*
- Sharma, R.S., Sharma, G.K., & Dhillon, G.P.S. (1996), Epidemiology & control of malaria in India, Govt. of India, *Min. of Health & Family Welfare,* National Malaria Eradication Programme.
- Sustaining Calcutta, *EIP Working Report* (1995), CMWSA, CMDA.
- Unpublished report on Malarial Incidence as found in Malaria Clinic of School of Tropical Medicine, 1998.

Chapter - 4

Mosquito Borne Diseases and Vector Diversity in Kolkata with Special Reference to Malaria

Sajal Bhattacharya* and Subhas Chandra Santra**

Abstract

Due to its involvement as a vector in diseases as debilitating as Malaria, Dengue, Filariasis, Chikungunya, Japanese Encephalitis (JE) and Yellow Fever (YF), mosquito is regarded as the numero uno public health enemy. All, but the last two, are endemic in Kolkata, where rapid urbanisation, coupled with deterioration of urban and peri-urban sanitation due to continuous population influx, contributed to new mosquitogenic environment. In view of the above prospectives, an attempt has been made to identify the mosquito vector diversity, through our study, with reference to Malaria, in the city and its suburbs. Persual of literature and an analysis of the incidence of Malaria cases, registered in the Calcutta Municipal Corporation (CMC) and Directorate of Health Services (Malaria) West Bengal between 1981 and 1996, reveal, that clinical manifestations of the infections were observed in all the years, encompassing all the three distinct seasons, with a pronounced peak in the rainy season (July to October).

Our collection recorded 18 species of mosquitoes, comprising of five genera, viz. Culex, Anopheles, Aedes, Armigeres and Mansonia. Amongst these, Culex (71.59%) topped the list, while Mansonia occupied the last position (0.86%). Armigeres, represented by Ar. subalbatus, showed a frequency of 6.61%. Anopheles, represented by 7 species, constituted 15.39% of the total catch, and atleast three (An. annularis, An. stephensi, An. subpictus complex) of them are malaria vectors in India. Cx. vishnui complex (8.54%), collected mainly from the adjoining suburbs of Kolkata,

---

* Department of Zoology and Post Graduate Department of Environmental Science, Asutosh College, Kolkata-700026, India.

** Department of Enviornmental Science, University of Kalyani, Nadia, India.

is a recognized vector of JE in India, and hence its prevalence is noteworthy. Aedes aegypti, a potential vector of Dengue and Yellow Fever, has also been registered during the study. Although, YF hasn't been reported to date in Kolkata (and India), yet the region is believed to be a "Yellow Fever receptive area".

Introduction

Amongst all the insect vectors of human disease, mosquito stands out as, by far, the most medically important fauna. It is responsible for the death and incalculable misery of millions of people every year, and is, therefore, the numero uno public health enemy (Chandler and Read, 1981). Mosquitoes have greatly affected the course of human events and continue to do so even today, thereby making a mockery of the repeated innovations in the technology that man adopts for their control. About 3500 species of mosquitoes have been identified all over the world (Schmidt and Roberts, 1996). There is considerable evidence for the resurgence of some mosquito-borne diseases. Malaria, for instance, has flared up in many countries, that formerly had it under control, and there have been almost world-wide epidemic of dengue, too. Two billion people, encompassing 102 countries, live in regions, where endemic malaria prevails, or, has reappeared. An estimated one hundred million infected individuals per year have been reported around the world, thereby contributing enormously to morbidity and mortality (Gentillini *et al.*, 1990, Breman, 1992).

In India, mosquito plays a major role for the transmission of more human diseases than any other group of arthropods. About 400 species of mosquitoes, belonging to 19 genera and 40 subgenera, are recorded from the country. Of these, only 4 genera, viz. Anopheles, Culex, Aedes and Mansonia, are vectors of various mosquito-borne diseases (Tewari, 1995). Major mosquito-borne diseases, reported in India, are Malaria, Filariasis, Dengue, Japanese Encephalitis, and Chikungunya. To date, 18 different arboviruses have been isolated, and identified from fourteen species and two species complexes of mosquitoes. Of these, three mosquito-borne viruses, viz. Japanese Encephalitis (JE), Dengue (four serotypes) and Chikungunya, are of major public health importance in our country (Reuben *et al.*, 1988). Malaria, Bancroftian filariasis, Dengue and Dengue haemorrhagic fever are endemic in Kolkata. In India, the first isolation of Chikungunya virus was made in Kolkata in 1963 (Shah *et al.*,

1964, Pavri *et al.*, 1964, Bhattacharya and Hati, 1986, Bhattacharya, 1996, Bhattacharya and Mukherjee, 1996). Rogers (1901) investigated the seasonal prevalence of *Anopheles and malaria fever in Lower Bengal. Covell (1932) had recorded 13 species of Anopheles in early 30s. These were Anopheles subpictus, An. vagus, An. ludlowii, An. stephensi, An. fuliginosus, An. pallidus, An. pseudojamesi, An. sinensis and An. barbirostris.* Although Covell has not mentioned about the other genera of mosquitoes, records show that sporadic mosquito faunastic surveys had been undertaken in between 1965 to 1987 in Kolkata and its adjoining areas (Ghosh and Hati, 1966, Das *et al.*, 1971, Mukhopadhyay and Hati, 1978 and Hati *et al.*, 1987). Pramanik *et al.* (1992) made a faunastic study in 1989-91 on mosquitoes in greater Kolkata and adjoining areas of the districts of 24-Parganas (North and South), Hooghly and Howrah. The different species of mosquitoes collected and identified during these surveys have been listed in Table-1.

Table - 1

Mosquito species reported from greater Kolkata and nearby suburbs during 1965-91.

1. *Aedes*

1.1 *Ae. aegypti*

1.2 *Ae. albopictus*

1.3 *Ae. vittatus*

2. *Anopheles*

2.1 *An. aitkenil sp. complex*

2.2 *An. annularis*

2.3 *An. barbirostris*

2.4 *An. culicifacies sp complex*

2.5 *An. jeyporiensis*

2.6 *An. kochi*

2.7 *An. majidi*

2.8 *An. aconitus*

2.9 *An. nigerrimus*

2.10 *An. stephensi*

2.11 *An. subpictus sp. complex*

2.12 *An. sundaicus*

2.13 *An. turkhudi*

2.14 *An. vagus*

3. *Armigeres*

3.1 *Ar. kuchingensis*

3.2 *Ar. subalbatus*

3.3 *Ar. theobaldi*

4. *Culex*

4.1 *Cx. bitaeniorhynchus*

4.2 *Cx. cornutus*

4.3 *Cx. epidesmus*

4.4 *Cx. gelidus*

4.5 *Cx. mimeticus*

4.6 *Cx. quinquefasciatus*

4.7 *Cx. sinensis*

4.8 *Cx. sitiens*

4.9 *Cx. tritaeniorhynchus*

4.10 *Cx. vishnui*

4.11 *Cx. whitmore*

5. *Mansonia*

5.1 *Ma. annulifera*

5.2 *Ma. indiana*

5.3 *Ma. uniformis*

6. *Toxorhynchites*

6.1 *To. splendens*

As a result of population growth, increasing urbanisation, and continuing pressure on scarce natural resources, the epidemiology of malaria, filariasis, dengue and encephalitis and their manifestations as a public health problem are undergoing profound modification indeed in several parts of the world, including India. Economic activity of man, in particular irrigation of new land areas, leading to the creation of a large number of artificial places, where mosquitoes may lay their eggs, also has a major impact in the prevalence of certain mosquito-borne diseases. WHO, (1993)

Rapid urbanisation and Industrialisation in Kolkata and its adjoining areas for the last few decades contributed to new mosquitogenic environment. Resurgence of *Plasmodium falciparum*, the causative agent of malignant malaria since early 1980s and their resistance to Chloroquine as well as spread of resistance to insecticides in the malaria vectors have made the malariogenic situations more complex (Bhattacharya *et al.*, 1996, Bhattacharya and Mukherjee 1996). For the last few decades no systematic and extensive study on mosquitoes, encompasing all the possible ecological zones of Kolkata and its adjoining areas has been done.

Retrospect of Mosquito Borne Diseases in Kolkata

Malaria

Malaria is endemic in Kolkata over 300 years back. Job Charnok landed here in 1690 with 1200 Englishmen amongst whom 460 died of malaria (O' Malley, 1914).

National Malaria control programme wae started in India in 1953. Malaria was almost controlled till early 1960s, but resurgence of the disease was reported again since early 1970s (Table - 7). In Kolkata, indigenous cases of falciparum malaria was, however not reported before 1981 (Dutta *et al.*, 1982). Yearly percentage of *P. falciparum* malaria against all malaria cases in Kolkata has been shown in Table - 2A and Table - 2B.

Table - 2A

Incidence of *Plasmodium falciparum* malaria amongst all malaria cases in Kolkata, West Bengal (1981-1989) (Bhattacharya *et al.* 1993)

	Kolkata		West Bengal	
Year	Number of *P. falciparum* cases	Percent of *P. falciparum* amongst all malaria cases	Number of *P. falciparum* cases	Percent of *P. falciparum* amongst all malaria cases
1981	21	0.35	2603	8.4
1982	15	0.22	4991	14.2
1983	333	1.74	4161	9.7
1984	1184	4.54	5780	12.5
1985	1667	9.26	10846	23.3
1986	898	5.71	14096	26.3
1987	613	3.77	9403	20.4
1988	633	3.70	5562	15.3
1989	718	4.5	6539	18.3

Source: Bhattacharya *et al.* (1993).

Table - 2B

Epidemiological Data on Malaria in West Bengal and Kolkata Municipal Corporation Area

Year	Blood slide examined	Total (+)ve	*Pf* cases	Deaths	ABER	*Pf*%	SPR
West Bengal							
1990	1610243	27531	3690	4	2.79	13.4	1.71
1991	1345197	40452	7771	13	3.19	19.2	2.17
1992	2159242	28179	7858	43	3.73	27.8	1.31
1993	2078000	46138	8723	37	3.40	18.9	2.2
1994	2535647	74293	15379	52	4.10	20.5	2.9
1995	2528000	91014	17226	87	4.0	18.9	3.6
1996	2172983	80127	15629	55	-	17.0	3.7
1997*	1302740	38795	4173	22			
Calcutta							
1990	76936	13624	552	0	2.0	0.7	17.7
1991	66854	15606	708	0	1.8	1.1	23.3
1992	82180	17969	728	0	2.2	0.9	21.8
1993	74161	19084	1802	3	1.5	2.4	25.6
1994	85815	18298	2283	7	2.2	2.7	21.3
1995	131000	36804	5725	52	2.9	4.4	28.1
1996	174000	44602	6467	17	3.9	14.5	25.6
1997*	77994	15719	1084	14			

* Provisional data upto September 1997

ABER = Annual Blood slide examination rate

SPR = Slide postivity rate

Pf = *Plasmodium falciparum*

Source: Mukhopadhyay *et al.* (1997)

Table - 7

Yearly Incidence of Malaria in India, West Bengal and Kolkata

	India			West Bengal			Kolkata		
Year	Total	*P.falciparum*	Death	Total	*P.falciparum*	Death	Total	*P.falciparum*	Death
1971	13222398			1006	54		46		
1972	1428649	142177		4181	386		187	1	
1973	1930373	265154		13603	3697		13		
1974	1367658	476922	3	18938	1838		519	2	
1975	5166142	722451	99	39634	7707		2071	2	
1976	6467215	753713	59	28917	1968		3150	3	
1977	4740900	459867	55	15722	168		1970	2	
1978	4144385	548567	74	12255	432		1278		
1979	3064697	558423	196	11296	665		2378	1	
1980	2896000	588011	207	22219	1733		2432	3	
1981	2666244	589596	170	30717	2603		6660	21	
1982	2182303	551057	187	34237	4991		6785	15	
1983	1895297	600964	239	41861	4161		19388	338	
1984	2184446	655545	247	46340	5780		26056	1184	
1985	1864380	545005	213	46510	10846		18201	1667	
1986	1792168	638276	323	53620	13131		15723	898	
1987	1647485	611588	188	46029	9403		16237	613	
1988	1850060	680000	209	36318	5562		17055	633	
1989	2020000	750000	268	35624	6484		16740	718	
1990	2020000	750000	353	27531	3690	4	13624	352	0
1991	2117460	690000	421	40452	7771	13	15606	708	0
1992	2130000	880000	422	28179	7858	43	17969	728	0
1993	2210000	850000	354	46138	8723	37	19084	1802	4
1994	2510000	990000	1422	74293	15379	52	18298	2283	7
1995	2930000	1140000	1151	91014	17226	87	36804	5725	52
1996	3035588	1179561	1010	80127	15629	55	44602	6467	17
1997	2660557	1007366	879	79881	11480	74	34514	5684	38
1998	2098356	914584	653	132088	25156	77(26)**	88402	16464	53(10)**
1999	1865874	882412	853	197259	57245	155(41)**	132367	37789	79(28)**

1999—Provisional ** unconfirmed

Source: Hati (2001).

Clinical manifestations of the infections were observed in all the three seasons, viz. summer, rainy (monsoon), and winter, and Malaria represents 9.57% of the total fever cases, with a peak in the rainy season (12.93%) (Bhattacharya and Mukherjee, 1996). These observations suggest that, there is perennial transmission of the disease, and fluctuations in the level of the circulation of the parasites in its maintenance cycle. For the last few decades, investigators have been referring *An. stephensi* as the only vector of malaria in Kolkata (Hati and Mukhopadhayay, 1980, Hati *et al.* 1987).

Filariasis

Kolkata is an endemic zone for Bancroftian filariasis (Bhattacharya and Hati, 1986). The causative agent of the disease is Wuchereria bancrofti. Culex quinquefasciatus, the principal vector of the disease, constitutes 97% of the nocturnal manbiting mosquitoes of Kolkata (Mukhopadhyay and Hati, 1978), and 4.6% of them were recorded previously to be the naturally infected in this area (Ghosh and Hati, 1966). In three years (1966-69), 9406 new patients and 74033 old patients attended the 'Filaria outdoor clinic of the School of Tropical Medicine, Kolkata. In 1984, the attendance of new cases was 2884 (female 1581 and male 1303). About 3,000 new cases are detected every year in the 'outdoor Filariasis Clinic' of the School of Tropical Medicine, Kolkata (Bhattacharya and Hati, 1986).

Dengue and Dengue Haemorrhagic fever (DHF)

Kolkata has long experience of recurrent outbreaks of dengue (Seal, 1981, Mukherjee *et al.*, 1987). A major outbreak of dengue fever with haemorrhagic manifestations (DHF) first occurred in Kolkata in 1963 (Sarkar *et al.*, 1967). DHF again broke out in Kolkata in October, 1990. Out of 55 Paediatric patients, 10 died. *Aedes aegypti* is the recognised vector (Gilotra and Bhattacharya, 1968, Biswas *et al.*, 1993).

Chikungunya

In India, the first isolation of Chinkungunya virus was made in Kolkata during an outbreak of haemorrhagic fever in July, 1963 (Shah *et al.*, 1964, Pavri *et al.*, 1964). All age-groups were affected, although the disease was more in children. Transmission of Dengue, DHF and Chinkungunya in Kolkata has been attributed to Aedes aegypti (Rao and Anderson, 1964, Gilotra and Bhattacharya, 1964, Sarkar *et al.*, 1964).

Keeping in view with the above perspectives, an attempt has been made to know the mosquito species composition, their seasonal variations, ecobehavioural patterns of the diurnal and nocturnal man-biting mosquitoes, vectorial status in relation to the epidemiology of the mosquito-borne diseases endemic in Kolkata. In the present communications, we report the data of the mosquito faunastic survey conducted during 20th June, 1993-27th May 1996. Besides, we reviewed the mosquito-vector-diversity and mosquito-borne diseases in Kolkata. This study will be helpful in formulating and implementing strategies for the containment of various mosquito vectors, and in turn the mosquito-borne diseases.

Materials and Methods

Study site

Kolkata is situated on the eastern bank of the river Hooghly, about 48 km. away from the Bay of Bengal. The soil is formed of alluvial deposits of the Gangetic delta, only approx. 5.3 m. above the sea level. Three meteorologically distinct seasons, a long summer characterised by intermittent rain fall (the premonsoon), an equally prominent monsoon, and a mild dry winter characterise its climate. According to 1991 Census, stable population of Kolkata is 10, 916, 272. If we add to the daily commuters, who spend their whole day here, the number of people, Kolkata has to accomodate, will be atleast another 3 million. According to UNFPA estimates, in the year 2000 A.D., Kolkata has become among, the ten most populated cities in the world (Bhattacharya *et al.*, 1985). The inhabitants of this cosmopolitan city has a diverse standard of living, from occupying the lavish and huge apartments to temporary hutments (the poverty-stricken ones).

Methodology

During our study, adult mosquitoes were collected from different places and biotopes, encompassing all the possible ecological zones, in Kolkata and adjoining areas with the help of aspirators and battery-operated torches. Mosquito collections were made between 6.00 a.m. and 7.00 a.m., and between 6.30 a.m. and 7.30 p.m., from Cattle sheds, human habitations, temporary hutments (jhupris). Attempts have also been made to collect adults from car-sheds of long distance trains and inter-state truck-terminals in Kolkata. Larvae were collected from drains, fields, ponds, artificial containers, and domestic reservoirs. They were brought to the Laboratory, and allowed to emerge into adults in mosquito-cages. Mosquitoes were also captured off human baits. Species identification was based on Christophers (1933), Barraud (1934), Wattal and Kalra (1961), and Hati (1979).

Observation and Discussion

Atleast 104 species of mosquitoes under ten different genera are recorded in Bengal since 1900 (Pramanik *et al.*, 1992). Atleast 35 species of mosquitoes were reported from greater Kolkata and its adjoining suburbs during 1965 to 1991. Our collection of three years in Kolkata and adjoining suburbs showed 18 species of mosquitoes comprising of five genera, viz. Culex, Anopheles, Aedes, Armigeres and Mansonia (Table - 3).

Table - 3

Mosquitoes Collected from Kolkata and Adjoining Suburbs During June 1993 to May, 1996

Name	Number	%
Anopheles annularis	617	3.38
An. barbirostris	69	0.37
An. culicifacies complex	87	0.47
An. hyrcanus complex	48	0.26
An. stephensi	551	3.02
An. subpictus	1012	5.55
An. vagus	419	2.30
Armigeres subalbatus	1205	6.61
Aedes aegypti	806	4.42
Ae. albopictus	201	1.10
Culex bitaeniorhynchus	89	0.48
Cx. gelidus	36	0.19
Cx. pseudovishnui	381	2.09
Cx. quinquefasaciatus	11352	62.35
Cx. tritaeniorhynchus	696	3.82
Cx. vishnui	479	2.63
Mansonia annulifera	62	0.34
Ma. indiana	95	0.52

Amongst these, Culex (71.59%) topped the list, while Mansonia occupied the last position (0.86%). The genus Armigeres, represented by Ar. subalbatus only, showed a frequency of 6.61%. The genus Anopheles, represented by 7 species, constituted 15.39% of the total catch, and atleast four (*An. annularis, An. stephensi, An. culicifacies* complex, *An. subpictus* complex) of them are malaria vectors in India (Rao, 1984, Panicker *et al.*, 1981, Kulkarni, 1983). *An. culicifacies* complex, mainly obtained from vacant coaches of long distance trains and drivers' cabins of inter-state trucks, was not reported in recent past from Kolkata, although it is a potential vector of malaria in many parts of India, including West Bengal. Further, it has been found in isolated pockets during the survey. No larva has been obtained in that period, and hence , in all probability, this species has not been ecologically establised, as yet, and must have been imported through trains, trucks and other such vehicles to Kolkata and its adjoining areas. Only a single *An. culicifacies* has been captured off human bait in the course of survey. *Cx. vishnui* complex (8.54%) was collected mainly from the adjoining suburbs of Kolkata. *Cx. tritaeniorhnchus* (44.73%) was predominant followed by *Cx. vishuni* (30.78%) and *Cx. pseudovishnui* (24.48%), Banerjee *et al.* (1995), also, obtained three members of the complex from Bidhannagar, adjacent to Kolkata.

Prevalence of *Cx. vishnui* complex is note-worthy, because they are the recognised vectors of JE in India (Reuben *et al.*, 1988). In West Bengal, JE virus has been isolated from *Cx. vishnui* (Hati & Bhattacharya, 1987). Presence of these mosquito species, along with the reservoirs/ amplifying hosts of JE - the pigs and some domestic and paradomestic birds (Bhattacharya *et al.*, 1986) in this area, necessitated the launching of a monitoring programme, although no cases of JE have been reported so far from Kolkata and its adjoining suburbs.

Presence of two species of Aedes also leads to an interesting inference. This type of mosquito is a favourite vector of dengue and yellow fever virus, although the latter disease is not reported to occur here, possibly because of the cross immunity conferred by other group - B arboviruses, whereby an "ecological barrier" is created (Park & Park, 1977); chances, however, exist that, the largely unvaccinated population of Kolkata (and India), congenial climatic conditions, and unchecked entry of travellers through aerial and maritime traffic may provide an ideal ground for its outbreak.

Of the 18,205 mosquitoes collected during the present study (Table-3), *Culex quinquefasciatus* was predominant with a frequency of 62.35%, followed by *Ar. subalbatus* (6.61%) and *An. subpictus* (5.55%). *Cx. gelidus* (0.19%) occupied the last position of the list. Amongst the seven anopheline species, *An. subpictus* (36.10%), *An. annularis* (22.01%), and *An. stephensi* (19.65%) occupied the first, second and third position, respectively. This observation on *An. subpictus* agrees with the finding of Chandra *et al.* (1994). *Aedes aegypti* (80.03%) was predominant amongst the Aedes mosquitoes. Altogether 15 species were captured off human baits in suburban Kolkata, while 7 species were registered in Kolkata (Table 4). Species , belonging to the genera Armigeres and Aedes, were predominantly daybiters, while all the Anophelese species were night-biters. *Cx. quinquefasciatus* was predominant of the total mosquitoes caught off human baits. Bhattacharya *et al.* (1982) reported, that, in West Bengal, most of the vector mosquitoes are not host - specific in the truest sense in their blood - sucking behaviour, and they take blood by chance rather than by choice. Several anopheline species previously considered as belonging to a single species are infact complexes of various sibling species, each of which has its own ecobehavioural characteristics (Bhattacharya, 1996). Cytogenetic studies of some vector species *viz. An. culicifacies, An. subpictus* and *An. stephensi* reveal that each of them consists of either 2, 3 or 4 biological forms / sibling species (Tandon *et al.*, 1995). For the last few decades, investigators have been referring *An. stephensi* as the only vector in Kolkata, albeit no attempt has so far been made to find out the existence of morphologically indistinguishable sibling species, if any, in the *An. stephensi* population in Kolkata (Bhattacharya & Mishra, 1995). Recently, we have started hybridization tests on *An. stephensi* in order to find out the existence of sibling species, if any. Owing to the existence of some recognised malaria vectors, *viz. An. annularis, An. subpictus* in Kolkata and adjoining areas, apprehension has been raised in certain quarters, that, besides *An. stephensi*, these species may have some role in the epidemiology of malaria, a disease which shows seasonal fluctuations (Tables-5 & 6). The data, presented here, corroborate the views of Bhattacharya and Mukherjee (1996) that there is perennial transmission of Malaria, and variations in the level of circulation of the malarial parasite in its maintenance cycle.

Table - 4

Mosquito Species Captured off Human Baits During the Study Period

Urban Kolkata	Suburban Kolkata
Culex quinquefasciatus	*Cx. quinquefasciatus*
Aedes aegypti	*Cx. vishnui*
Anopheles stephensi	*Cx. pseudovishnui*
An. subpictus	*Cx. tritaeniorhynchus*
An. vagus	*Ae. albopictus*
An. annularis	*Ae. aegypti*
Armigeres subalbatus	*An. annularis*
	An. stephensi
	An. hyrcanus complex
	An. barbiorstris
	An. subpictus
	An. vagus
	An. culicifacies
	Ar. subalbatus
	Mansonia indiana

Table - 5

Month-Wise Incidence of Malaria During 1981 to 1988 in Kolkata

Month	1981	1982	1983	1984	1985	1986	1987	1988	Sub total	%
Jan.	84	124	185	207	214	489	319	254	1878	1.49
Feb.	86	187	223	217	495	464	299	302	2273	1.80
Mar.	385	275	434	279	514	592	606	122	3207	2.55
Apr.	715	356	673	1414	1303	977	957	942	7337	5.82
May.	716	441	1015	2277	1191	1155	1044	1457	9296	7.38
Jun.	789	820	1432	2255	2474	995	1351	1701	11817	9.38
Jul.	730	1022	2574	4173	1871	1909	1644	2174	16097	12.7
Aug.	918	1020	3243	4750	2533	3421	2527	3350	21762	17.27
Sep.	875	1276	3617	3226	2708	1987	3469	2981	20139	15.98
Oct.	695	639	3205	2829	2500	1751	1991	2140	15750	12.50
Nov.	501	474	2082	2384	1378	1309	1531	1122	10781	8.56
Dec.	166	151	732	2045	856	565	599	540	5654	4.49
Grand Total									**125991**	

Source: Directorate of Health Services, Govt. of West Bengal (Malaria), Calcutta.

Table - 6

Month-wise Malariogical Data of An area of Kolkata (1995 and 1996)

			1995			*An. stephensi*	
Year/ Month	**Total slide examined**	**Total (+)ve**	**SPR**	**Total *Pf***	***Pf*%**	**Container index**	**Breteau index**
Jan	140	61	43.5	41	67.2	10	10
Feb	108	75	69.4	34	45.3	12.6	12
Mar	131	89	67.9	35	39.3	13	11
Apr	153	94	61.4	12	12.7	10	10
May	248	159	64.1	3	1.8	8.2	8
Jun	322	184	57.1	1	0.5	8.8	8
Jul	533	307	57.5	35	9.7	10	9
Aug	1129	531	47.0	71	13.3	7.8	8
Sep	778	381	48.9	14	3.6	9.2	9
Oct	750	392	52.2	110	28.0	12.5	12
Nov	1225	630	51.4	451	71.5	14	12
Dec	776	301	38.8	248	82.3	12.2	12
			1996				
Jan	330	107	32.4	54	50.4	2	2
Feb	218	60	27.5	27	45.0	2.2	2
Mar	96	32	3303	1	3.1	7.5	5
Apr	178	72	40.4	1	1.3	10	8
May	252	123	48.8	5	4.0	12.2	9
Jun	318	127	39.9	8	6.2	10.9	10
Jul	747	320	42.8	11	3.4	12.5	12
Total	**8432**	**4045**	**47.97**	**1162**	**28.72**		

Source : Mukhopadhyay *et al.* (1997).

Alteration of host parasite relationship, addition and alteration of mosquito vectors, and vectorial capacity may have some role in the present malaria situation in West Bengal (Bhattacharya *et al.*, 1993). In a given ecological stratum, the stability and complexity of mosquito-borne disease transmission increases with the increasing diversity of the vectorial system.

Our apprehension of multi-vectorial involvement in Malaria epidemiology in Kolkata is further reinforced by the study of Chakraborty and Tandon (1995), who opined, that, *An. Stephensi*, " The principle vector of malaria in the metropolis (Kolkata) is zoophilic and prefers to feed on bovine blood irrespective of the biotope and availability of the host." Study along this direction is necessary for a meaningful and target specific control of Malaria.

Acknowledgements

The authors remain grateful to Principal, Asutosh College, Kolkata, for extending all facilities for the work.

They also express their deep sense of gratitude to Professor A. K. Hati, former Director, school of Tropical Medicine, Kolkata, for his kind suggestion during the investigation.

Thanks are due to those students of Bio-science Faculty, Asutosh College, who have extended their help in carrying out the present work.

References

- Banerjee, A., Basu, D., Paul, A. K., Hati, A. K. (1995) Seasonal variation in mosquito fauna diversity in the newly built Township of Bidhannagar. *Abstract Book*, p-49. National Symoposium on perspectives in Biodiversity held in Indian Inst. of Chemical Biology, Calcutta, March 24-25.
- Barraud, P. J. (1934) *The fauna of British India including Ceylone and Burmah.* Vol. 5. Taylor & Francis, London p. 463.
- Bhattacharya, S., Chakraborty, S. , Mitra, A.K., Ghosh, K. K., Das, S., Chakraborty, M. S., Chatterjee, Arati, and Hati, A. K. (1982) Blood Meal Analysis of Certain Species of Mosquitoes of rural West Bengal. *Bull Cal. Sch. Trop. Med.* **30**: (2) - 43-45.
- Bhattacharya, S., Chakraborty, S. K., Chakraborty, S., Ghosh, K. K., Palit, A., Mukherjee, K. K. , Chakraborty, M. S., Tandon, N., and Hati, A. K. (1986) Density of Culex vishnui and appearance JE anti body in sentinel chicks and wild birds in relation to JE cases. *Tropical and Geographical Medicine.* 38 : 46-50

- Bhattacharya, S., (1985) Public Participation in the programme of mosquito control operation, *Proceedings of the seminar on urban Mosquitoes* held in Institute of Urban Management. The Calcutta Municipal Corporation, 29th August.
- Bhattacharya, S. and Mishra, B. (1995) Vector diversity in Malaria epidemiology. Abstract Book, page 21, *National Symposium on perspectives in Bio-diversity* held in Ind. Inst. of Chemical Biology, Calcutta, March 24-25.
- Bhattacharya, S. (1996) Vector diversity in Malaria epidemiology with special reference to Calcutta. *Abstract Book,* Xth European Meeting of the society for Vector Ecology held in Strasbourg, France, 2-6 September.
- Bhattacharya, S., Saha, S.K., Mukherjee, K. C. (1996) Epidemiological studies of malaria in relation to vectors in Calcutta. *Abstract Book,* XXth International Congress of Entomology held in Firenze, Italy, 25-31 August.
- Bhattacharya, S. and Mukherjee, K. C. (1996) Epidemiological studies of malaria in an endemic area of India. *Abstract Book,* p. 182. XIVth International Congress for Tropical Medicine and malaria, Nagasaki, Japan, 17-22 November.
- Bhattacharya, J., Mukherjee, H., Banerjee, A., and Hati, A. K. (1993) Recent studies on Plasmodium falciparum in West Bengal. *Your health.* **42**(11 and 12) 139-141.
- Bhattacharya, S. (1996) Cytogenetic diversity in the Malaria Vectorial system. *Abstract book.* National seminar on genes and genetic counselling held in BITM/Calcutta, 5th October.
- Bhattacharya, S. and Hati, A. K. (1986) Man - Culex quinquefasciatus contact in relation to transmission dynamics of Bancroftian filariasis. VIth International Congress of parasistology held in Brisbane, Australia, 24-31 August.
- Biswas, D., Dey, S., Dutta, R. N., and Hati, A. K. (1993) observation on the breeding habitats of Aedes aegypti in Calcutta following an episode of Dengue haemorrhagic fever. *Ind. Journal Med. Res (A)* **97** : 44-46.
- Breman, J.G. (1992) Malaria in the 1990-s. Perspectives, strategies and actions. *Abstract book.* No. 199, p. 55. 5th International Congress for Infectious diseases, held in Nairobi, Kenya, 7-11 June.
- Chandler, A. C. and Read, C.P. (1981) *Introduction to parasitology,* John Wiley and sons, Inc., New York, p. 822.
- Chakroborty, S. and Tandon, N. (1995) studies on host-preference of Anopheles stephensi in two ecological biotopes in calcutta metropolis. *Bull. Cal. Soh. Trop. Med.* **43** : (1-4): 11-12.
- Chandra, G., Chatterjee, S. N., Chatterjee, K. K., and Hati, A.K. (1994) Anophelines in an urban and a rural area of West Bengal. *Bull. Cal. Sch. Trop. Med.* **42** : (1) : 14-15.

- Christophers, S.R. (1933) *The fauna of British India* including Ceylone and Burmah, vol. 4, Taylor and Francis, London, p. 371.
- Covell, G. (1932) Malaria in Calcutta : *Records of Malaria, Survey of India*, **3** : 1-82.
- Das, U. P., Hati, A.K., Chaudhury, A.B. (1971) Nocturnal manbiting mosquitoes of urban and rural areas. *Bull. Cal. Sch. Trop. Med.* **19** : 80-83.
- Dutta, A., Mallick, K. K., Hati, A. K., and Mitra, S. B. (1982) Resurgence of Plasmodium falciparum malaria in Calcutta. *J. Ind. Med. Asson.*, **78** : 201-202.
- Gentillini, M., Danis, M., and Mouchet, J. (1990) Current strategies for the prevention of malaria, *Bull. Acad. Natl. Med.* **174 (1)** : 147-158 (Cited in WHO Quarterly Bibliography of Major Tropical Diseases 1990 Vol. 13, No. 3, p. 79.)
- Ghosh, S. M. and Hati, A. K. (1966), House frequenting mosquitoes of West Bengal and Calcutta : Detection of Filarial parasites in Anopheles and Culex sp., *Bull. Cal. Sch. Trop. Med.* **14** : 9-10.
- Gilotra, S. K. and Bhattacharya, N. C. (1968) Mosquito vectors of Dengue, Chikungunya Viruses in a rural area near Calcutta, *Bull. Cal. Sch. Trop. Med.* **16** : 41.
- Hati, A. K. (2001) *Medical Entomology*. Allied Book Agency, Calcutta. p. 201.
- Hati, A. K. (1979) *Medical Entomology*. Allied Book Agency, Calcutta. p. 140.
- Hati, A. K. and Bhattacharya, S. (1987). Biosystematics of Culex Vishnui and Culex pseudovishnui based on ecobehavioural pattern. *Proc. Ind. Acad. Sci.* (Animal sci.) **96** : 629-636.
- Hati, A. K., and Mukhopadhyay, A. K. ,(1980). Bionomics of Anopheles stephensi in Calcutta. *Proceedings of the Xth International Congress on Tropical Medicine and Malaria*. Phillippines, 9-15 November.
- Hati, A. K., Chatterjee, K. K., and Biswas, D. (1987). Day time resting habitats of Anopheles stephensi in an area of Calcutta. *Ind. J. Mal.* **24** : 85-87.
- Kulkarni, S. M. (1983) Detection of sporozoites in Anopheles subpictus in Bastar Districts, Madhya Pradesh. *Ind. J. Mal.* **20** : 159-160.
- Mukherjee, K. K., Chakraborty, S. K., P.N., Dey, S., and Chakraborty, M. S. (1987) out break of Febrile illness due to Dengue virus type - 3 in Calcutta during 1983. *Trans. R. Soc. Med. Hyz.* **81** : 1008.
- Mukhopadhyay, A. K., Karmakar, P, Hati, A.K and Dey, P. (1997) Recent Epidemiological status of Malaria in Calcutta Muncipal Corporation Area, *West Bengal Ind. Journal*. Malariology **34**: 188-196.
- Mukhopadhyay, A. K. and Hati, A. K. (1978) Man biting activity of Anopheles stephensi in Calcutta, *Bull. Cal. Sch. Trop. Med.* **26** : 5-7.
- O'Malley, L.S.S (1914). *Bengal District Gazetteer*. 24-Parganas District. Beng. Sec. Book. Dept. Calcutta.

- Panicker, K. N., Getta Bai, M., Bheem Rao, U. S. , Viswan, K., and Suryanarayanamurthy, K. (1981). An. subpictus, vector of malaria in coastal villages of South India. *Current Science* **50** : 694-695.
- Park, J. E. and Park, K. (1977), *Text book of Preventive And Social Medicine.* Banarsidas Bhanot Publishers, Jabalpur, India, pp. 758.
- Pavri, K. M., Banerjee, G., Anderson, C. R., Aikat. B. K. (1964) : Virological and serological studies of cases of haemorrhagic fever in Calcutta, materials collected by the Institute of Post Graduate Medical Education and Research (IPGME) Calcutta *Ind. J. Med. Res.* **52** : 692-697.
- Pramanik, M. K., Acharya, P. M. R., Ghosh, S., and Dutta Gupta, A. K. (1992). Mosquito Fauna of West Bengal. *Proc Zool. Soc.* (Suppl. : A) : 555-561.
- Rao, T. R. and Anderson, C. R. (1964). Concluding review on the papers on the out break of febrile illness with haemorrhagic manifestations in Calcutta. *Ind. J. Med. Res.* **52** : 727.
- Rao, T. R. (1984). *The Anophelines of India.* ICMR, New Delhi. pp. 538.
- Reuben, R., Kaul, H. N., and Soman, R. S. (1988) Mosquitoes of arboviral importance in India. *Mosquito borne diseases bulletin* vol. 5 No. S. 3-4 October - December, 1988. pp. 48-54.
- Rogers, L. (1901). The Seasonal prevalence of Anopheles and Malaria fever in lower Bengal and the practical application of the Mosquito theory. *J. Hyg. Camb.* 1 : 407-421.
- Sarkar, J. K., Chatterjee, S. N., and Chakraborty, S. K. (1964). Haemorrhagic fever in Calcutta : some epidemological observations. *Ind. J. Med. Res.* **52** : 651-659.
- Sarkar, J. K., Chatterjee, S. N., and Chakraborty, S. K. (1967). Three years study of mosquito borne haemorrhagic fever in Calcutta. *Trans. R. Soc. Trop. Med. Hyg.*,(**61**)725.
- Schmidt, G. D. and Roberts, L. S. (1996). *Foundations of Parasitology,* Wm. C. Brown Publishers, Dubuque IA, USA, p. 659.
- Seal, S. C. (1981) Epidemiology of Dengue and Haemorrhagic fever. *Bull. Cal. Sch. Trop. Med.* **29** : 106.
- Shah, K. V., Gilotra, S. K., Gibbs, C. J. (Jr.), and Rozeboom, I. E. (1964). Laboratory studies of transmission of Chikungunya virus by Mosquitoes, a preliminary report. *Ind. J. Med. Res.* **52** : 703-709.
- Tandon, N., Chakraborty, S., and Tandon, S. K. (1995). Biodiversity in Malaria vectors : An analysis. *Abstract Book,* pp. 39, National Symposium on perspectives in Biodiversity held in Indian Ins. of Chemical Biology. Calcutta, 24-25 March.
- Tewari, S. C. (1995) Mosquitoes of medical importance in Andaman and Nicobar Island. *Proceedings of the International Symposium on Vector Borne Diseases* National Academy of Vector Borne Diseases. Regional Medical Research Centre (I. C. M. R.). Bhubaneswer. India, pp. 91-97.

- Wattal, B. L. and Kalra, N. L. (1961). Regionwise pictorial keys to the female Indian Anopheles. *Bull Nath. Soc. Ind. Malar. Mosq. Dis.* **9** : 85-138.
- World Health Organization (1993). *A global strategy for malaria control.* WHO, Geneva, Switzerland, p. 30.

Chapter - 5

Vector Spectre: Pervention is the Cure

** Debashis Biswas*

Abstract

Mosquito borne maladies are on step rise around the world. Neither chemical nor bio-control agents alone can help tide over the crisis. What instead is solely needed now is to launch an integrated attack, for which entomologists have to be directly involved in fighting the battle. But is it possible in a country like India where policy makers are yet to crack the shell of their lackadaisical attitude towards mosquito abatement?

Introduction

Mosquitoes are deceptively dangerous. The world's leading disease carriers, they transmit 90 per cent of all insect - borne ailments and yet their size tends to instill an overconfidence in people for the simple reason that they can so easily be killed in large numbers through the use of chemicals or other devices. This overconfidence, in fact, is among the well documented reasons why malaria and other mosquito - borne maladies are increasing at an alarming pace around the world.

About malaria Around 2400 million people in 90 countries now is at risk of its infection. A staggering 500 million people suffer every year, of whom 2.7 million die, according to a report of the World Health Orgnisation (WHO, 1997). Nearly one-third of the global deaths occur among children below five. Over the past one - and - half decades, this hydra - headed monster has killed about 10 times as many children as all wars combined have in that period. The most startling point is that as a sequel to global warming, entomologists envisage that hitherto malaria - free places like the southern United States of America and southern Europe will become conducive to the spawning of mosquitoes, as a result of

* The Kolkata Muncipal Corporation, 149 A.J.C Bose Road, Kolkata-700094.

which an estimated 80 million fresh cases of malaria will occur there annually at end of the current century (Kristof, 1997).

Among the South-East Asian countries, the worst affected is India, accounting for more than 60 per cent of the total cases (Lal *et al.*, 1999). Officially, on an average 2.4 million Indians now suffer every year, 60 per cent of the cases being vivax, the rest falciparum and the number of deaths stands are around 750 per year. Back in the 1970s, the annual incidence of falciparum malaria in India was 13 per cent. It rose to 29.4 per cent in the 1980s. In the 1990s, the figure shot up to a whopping 41 per cent, suggesting that the scenario is getting grimmer by the day, despite the government's best efforts. Not only the cases of dreaded malaria, the death toll from it is on a steep rise. The official statistics - that tend to obfuscate reality - show that between 1974 to 1999, a total of 10,163 people succumbed to falciparum malaria: 488 during 1974 to 1979; 2,251 in the 1980s and 7,424 in the 1990s (Report from the Joint Director [Entomologist]).

The scenario of classical dengue as well as dengue haemorrhagic fever - both are viral diseases transmitted by *Aedes aegypti* - is no less frightening. They occur mainly among the urban communities in South-East Asia, the Eastern Mediterranean and the Americas. Roughly 100 million people suffer and several thousands die every year; and a population of an astonishing 2.5 billion in 100 countries is at risk (Director General of Health Services, 2000).

In some countries of South-East Asia and the Western Pacific, DHF - the fatal variety of dengue - has become the main cause of paediatric hospitalisation and a major cause of death among young children.

In India so far, 70 epidemics of dengue/ dengue haemorrhagic fever have occurred since the 1960s. Barring 2 or 3 states, the entire country is endemic for dengue. During 1996 to 1999, a total of 18,697 people contracted the ailment, of whom 617 died. About 70 per cent of the deaths occurred in Delhi. More annoyingly, once considered an urban problem, dengue has started to attack rural people too (Bhattacharya *et al.*, 1997).

In the countries of Central and South *America* and the *Caribbean*, around 160,000 cases occur every year, 2.6 per cent of which are DHF. A survey by the Pan American Health Organisation, reported in *Public Health,* has revealed that in the Americas, cases of dengue, including DHF, increased from 66,011 in 1980 to 276,758 in 1996.

Most importantly, the continental countries of South and Central America - where dengue and DHF were absent only a few years ago are now witnessing large-scale epidemics. Not a single continental Latin American country is currently free from dengue (Schmunis, 1998).

Entomologists envisage that the increased threat of dengue across the world is partly due to the widespread increase in urbanisation and construction, that provides ideal breeding sites of *Aedes aegypti.*

Lymphatic filariasis caused by three types of white, slender worms - *Wuchereria bancrofti, Brugia malayi* and *B. timori,* is another ailment posing a serious health problem, especially in the tropical countries where an estimated 751 million people are now exposed to its infection. In India, about 454 million people have a chance of becoming infected. Roughly 27 million people are harbouring microfilaria, of whom nearly 800,000 patients have already developed symptoms of the ailment (Sharma, 2000). Since filariasis is not killer disease, it never occupies newspaper headlines nor do the general public bother about it. But what a troublesome problem it is! In case of delayed treatment, an agonising symptom called elephantitis develops in different parts of the body, more particularly in the legs and scortum. For this, the patient becomes crippled physically as well as mentally and continues to remain so throughout life.

The deadliest of all insect-borne diseases is Japanese encephalitis spread mainly by three species of Culex - *C. vishmui, C. pseudovishnui* and *C. triteaniorhynchus* (Director General of Health Service, 2000). The rural populations in Japan and the South-East Asian countries - that live in huts close to paddy fields (the main breeding sites of the vectors) and rear pigs (the amplifiers of the JE virus)- mainly suffer the brunt. Strangely, it has unveiled its ugly face in Siberia too, the North-East part of Russia which remains covered with ice more than half the year (Manson-Bahr and Bell, 1987).

In India, J.E. made its debut in vellore in September, 1955 (Carey *et al.*, 1969) - but its outbreak in an epidemic form first occurred in West Bengal in June, 1973 (Chakraborty *et al.*, 1975). As revealed by a survey of the directorate of National Anti Malaria Programme (Director General of Health Service, 2000), as many as 10 states of the country are now highly endemic for J.E. and these are : Uttar Pradesh, Assam, Andhra Pradesh, Bihar, Goa, Haryana,

Karnataka, Manipur, Tamil Nadu and and West Bengal. During 1978 to April 2000, more than 79 thousand people in these states got the infection and 35 per cent of them died.

For curbing such ailments, early diagnosis and proper case managment apart, abatement of the offending mosquitoes too is equally important. But how is this possible in a country like India where people, including political leaders by and large do not have an orientation of the subject nor there is any governmental initiative to involve entomologists in planning and implementing vector control stategies?

Many people are still inclined to believe that insecticidal spraying will help them to tide over the crisis. They are mistaken. Contrary to public perception, the battle cannot be won by spraying insecticides. Having been under indiscriminate threats from various insecticides for decades, the tiny tormentors have strategically more evolved than ever before, proving themselves enormously adaptable to new threats and environments.

The story of the yet-to-be-won fight began in the 1950s. With the advent of DDT (dichloro diphenyl trichloroethane)- a highly effective organochlorine insecticide, a new era of mosquito-bashing ushered in. The earlier practice of eliminating or modifying spawning sites and reducing man-vector contact both by environmental management measures - was replaced by a single method: spraying the walls and ceilings of houses in malaria prone areas with DDT. Initially, this method produced very impressive results. So, in 1957, the World Health Orgnisation set up a worldwide programme of malaria eradiction.

India and Sri Lanka provided good examples of what could be achieved. The number of cases in India slumped from 75 million with 0.8 million deaths in 1951 to only 50 thousand with no deaths in 1961. Sri Lanka with 3 million cases in1947 had only 29 in 1964. People heaved a sigh of relief (Hati, 1979).

Overwhelmed by the results, many people thought malaria had been wiped out and that there would be no further resurgence of this malady in this country and outside. Thus began the slackening of the anti-malarial programme. But the euphoria did not last long. With the development of DDT-resistance among many species of vector mosquitoes in different parts of the world, the people's over enthusiasm evaporated. Bewildered, people resorted to indoor spraying by other insecticides such as BHC, dieldrin, malathion etc. Unfortunately, they too lost their efficacy at some point of time (WHO, 1992).

Going by the reports in India, organochlorine, weapons (DDT, BHC, HCH) are futile, organophosphorus insecticide malathion is useless, especially against *Anopheles stephensi* and *An. culififacies* - the prime vectors of urban and rural malaria respectively (Nagpal and Sharma, 1995) - as is fogging with pyrethrum - an extract from the petals of a common variety of *Chandramallika* flower (*Chrysanthemum cinerariaefolium)* (Chakraborty, 2000). Why? Because the smoke repels the mosquito but does not kill it. Besides, the insects. *An. stephensi* for an instance, now rests outdoors instead of indoors (Hati *et al.*, 1988; Hati, 1997). Propoxur, a carbamate compound too has lost its credibility against *An. stephensi,* more particularly in Kolkata, thanks to its indiscriminate use by private pest control agencies and city dwellers (Mukhopadhyay *et al.*, 1996). Research reveals that repellents commonly used by all sectors of people are no longer effective, which is why repellent users suffer from malaria to the extent of 80 to 85 per cent, while those employ bednets hardly suffer (only 3 to 4 per cent). Clearly starting that mats and coils are not the answer (Biswas, 2000).

For reducing man-vector contact, the latest idea is to use insecticide-more precisely mosquito nets treated with synthetic pyrethroid (deltamethrin, permethrin, cyfluthrin or lambda-cyhalothrin) (Chavasse *et al.*, 1999). But in cities like Kolkata, where most people do not even use traditional mosquito nets for the lack of space or merely reluctancy, will ITNs ever make any sense? Or will such nets be effective in areas like Assam, Papua New Guinea and Cambodia, where malaria bearing mosquitoes are completely exophilic and exophagic (Reuben, 1995; WHO, 2000).

Besides developing resistance to insecticides, many species of vectors have changed their resting habits to bypass the danger. An instance from Kolkata : in this metropolis, *An. stephensi* once used to rest indoors but now do so at outdoor. They enter bedrooms only when they need blood that necessary to nourish their eggs. This phenomenal change, is presumably due to the excitorepellatory impact of DDT used in this city during the national malaria eradication programme in the 1950s and 1960s (Hati *et al.*, 1988). Situation is like, taming the tiny terrorists by indoor spraying - no matter how powerful the insecticide - is impossible.

Like adults, larvae too have grown smarter and can now easily digest many larvicides. In Kolkata, once considered so suitable for their destruction, temephos is of no use today, especially against *An. stephensi* larvae (Hati, 1979; Chakraborty and Tandon, 2002).

The role of fish (guppy, gambusia etc.) too is now increasingly becoming fishy, especially in the cities for genuine reasons of excessive water pollution and clogging of surface drains, ditches, canals and other breeding sites.

Some people's enthusiasm about the killing of mosquito larvae by newly developed ecofriendly bacterial toxins is also fast waning, and here is the reason : a study reportedly in *Current Science* (Adak *et al.*, 1995), has revealed that the larvae of *Culex quinquefasciatus,* that predominating in India and many other countries, can show grow 150 - fold resistant to the toxin of *Bacillus sphaericus* following 20 to 25 rounds of its application within a year, thereby suggesting that such a toxin cannot be the weapon of choice for a long-term containment programme of *C. quinquefasciatus* larvae. Besides it has a very low efficacy against the larvae of *Aedes aegypti,* the prime vector of dengue DHF and YF.

The last missile left in our store is the toxin of *Bacillus thuringiensis* var. *isralliensis.* But this too has some limitations. Its action in dirty water lasts hardly for a week. So the larve of *C. quinquefasciatus* and other dirty water breeders cannot be destroyed by using it on a regular basis (Biswas *et al.*, 1997). The reason as explained by J. Margalit and D. Dean (Margalit and Dean, 1985) is : In places such as open drains, roadside gullies, abandoned ponds, ditches, canals and unused wells, the toxin of *B.t.i.* cannot yield desired results because of its rapid biodegradation caused by water pollution as well as its adsorption on organic particles. The toxin instead has to be used for killing mosquito larvae only in fresh water collections. Sprayed at the rate of 0.5 to 1 gram per square meter of a breeding site at fortnightly intervals, this toxin will substantially control the menace of malaria bearing mosquitoes (Pal and Tandon, 2001; Kumar *et al.*, 1995).

Scientists working in the field of mosquito control now realise that neither that chemical insecticides nor biochemical agents alone can bring a magic bullet solution. What instead is solely needed is an intergrated attack, more precisely, an area specific strategy for mosquito abatement(ASSMA), involving judicious use of effective, less polluting insecticides, biocontrol measures; environmental management practices; information, education and communication activities; and enforcement of legal steps to involve people in removing mosquitogenic conditions from their houses and neighbourhoods. A superb proposition! But how can this ASSMA be planned and implemented in this country where entomologists have not yet been involved in fighting the battle?

In 1995, the Directorate of NMEP brought out a *Manual for Malaria Action Programme (MAP),* wherein it has been stated that for planning and implementing vector control strategies there must be a biologist (entomologist) for every 25.6 square kilometers in malaria prone city (Directorate General of Health Services, 1995). Unfortunately, for reasons best known to them, most of the state government in India are yet to through this Namp - prescription. It is distressing to hear that the entomological activities in almost all states of the country have long been running without entomologists. Cooking without a cook ! How bad !

References

A report from the Joint Director (Entomologist), Regional office for Health & Family Welfare, Govt. of India, Kolkata.

- Adak, T., Mittal, P. K., Raghavendra, K., Subbarao, S. K., Ansari, M. A. & Sharma, V. P. (1995). Resistance to *Bacillus sphaericus* in *C. quinquefasciatus* Say 1823. *Current Science,* **69(8)** : 695-698.
- Bhattacharya, N., Neogi, D. K., Hati, A. K., Pramanik, N. Banerjee, A. & Mukherjee, K. K. (1997). An outbreak of dengue fever in rural area of West Bengal. *Ind. J. Med. Microbiol.,* **15 (3)** : 139-141.
- Biswas, D. (2000). Virulent resurgence of malaria in Calcutta, West Bengal. *J. Ind. Med. Assoc.,* **98(10)** : 638-643.
- Biswas, D., Ghosh, S. K., Dutta, R. N. & Mukherjee, A. K. (1997). Field trial of Bacticide on larval population of two species of vector mosquitoes in Calcutta. *Ind. J. Malariol.,* **34 (1)** : 37-41
- Carey, D.E., Myers, R.M., Reuben, R. & Webb, J.K.C. (1969). Japanese encephalitis in South India : a summary of recent knowledge. *J. Ind. Med. Assoc.,* **52** : 10-15.
- Chakraborty, P. K. (2000). Guidelines on vector control by insecticide fogging under National Anti Malaria Programme. Go. No. 4-6/97-98/ NMEP (St). *Fogging - Mal.,* Govt. of India, Ministry of Health and Family Welfare, Dept. of Health, January 21.
- Chakraborty, S. K., Sarkar, J.K., Chakraborty, M. S., Mukherjee, M. K., Mukherjee, K. K., Das, B. C. & Hati, A. K. (1975). The first epidemic of Japanese encephalitis studied in India - virological studies. *Ind. J. Med. Res.,* **63** : 77-82.
- Chakroborty, S. & Tandon, N. (2002). Insecticide susceptibility status of *Anopheles stephensi* (Liston) in Calcutta, West Bengal. *Ind. J. Malariol.* (In press).

- Chavasse, D., Reed, C. & Attawell, K. (1999). *Insecticide Treated Net Projects : A Handbook for Managers* published by Malaria Consorthium, London School of Hygiene & Tropical Medicine and Liverpool School of Tropical Medicine, UK.
- Directorate General of Health services, Ministry of Health Services and Family Welfare, Govt. of India, Delhi (1995). *Operational Manual for Malaria Action Programme (MAP)*, pp : 63-64.
- Hati, A. K. (1979). *Medical Entomology* published by Allied Book Agency, Kolkata.
- Hati, A. K. (1997). Urban malaria vector biology. *Ind. J. Med. Res.*, **106** : 195-208.
- Hati, A. K., Chatterjee, K. K., Biswas, D., Mukherjee, A. K. & Saha, D. (1988). A newly discovered habitat of *Anopheles stephensi* in present day Calcutta with evidence of natural malaria infection. *Tropical & Geographical Medicine* (Switzerland), **40 (4)** : 376-377.
- Kristof, N. D. (1997). Malaria makes a comeback, and is more deadly than before. *The New York Times,* January 8.
- Kumar, A. Sharma, V. P., Thavasclvam, D. & Sumodan, P. K. (1995). Control of *Anopheles stephensi* breeding in construction sites and abandoned overhead tanks with *Bacillus thuringiensis* var. *israelensis. J. Amer. Mosq. Contr. Assoc.,* **11(1)** : 86-89.
- Lal, S., Dhillon, G.P.S. & Aggarwal, C.S. (1999). Epidemiology and control of malaria *Ind. J. Pediatr.,* **66** : 547-554.
- Manson-Bahr, P.E.C. & Bell, D. R. (1987). *Manson's Tropical Diseases,* nineteenth edition.
- Margalit, J. Dean, D. (1985). The story of *Bacillus thuringiensis* var. *israelensis., J. Amer. Mosq. Contr. Assoc.,* **1(1)** : 1-7.
- Mukhopadhyay, A. K., Chakroborty, S., Karmakar, P. K. & Banerjee, P. (1996). Insecticidal susceptibility status of *Anopheles stephensi* Liston in selected areas of Calcutta, West Bengal. *Ind. J. Pub. Health,* **40(4)** : 130-132.
- Nagpal, B. N. & Sharma, V. P. (1995). *Indian Anophelines* published by Oxford & IBH Publishing Co. Pvt. Ltd.
- National Institute of Communicable Diseases, Directorate General of Health Services, Govt. of India (2000), Dengue/ Dengue haemorrhagic fever : calls for an immediate public health action. *CD Alert,* **4 (4)** : 1-8.
- National Institute of Communicable Diseases, Directorate General of Health Services, Govt. of India (2000). Japanese encephalitis. *CD Alert,* **4 (3)** : 1-8.
- Pal, M. K. & Tandon, N. (2001). Field evaluation of *Bacillus thuringiensis* var *israelensis* (Bacticide) against *Anopheles stephensi* breeding in Calcutta city, *J. Commun. Dis.,* **33 (2)** : 143-146.

- Reuben, R. (1995). Pyrethroid impregnated bednets and curtains for control of malaria and other vector - borne disease. *NAV News Letter* (published by the National Academy of Vector Borne Diseases) **1** : 1-2.
- Schmunis, G. A. (1998). Dengue in the Americas. *Public Health,* **14** : 8-16.
- Sharma, R. C. (2000). Lecture note on lymphatic filariasis distributed among the traunees of the WHO - sponsored *9th training course on vector biology and control,* held at the NICD., New Delhi, October 5-29, 2000.
- WHO (1992). Fifteenth report of the WHO expert committee on vector biology and control. *WHO. Tech. Rep. Ser.,* **818** : 1-58.
- WHO (1997). *Tropical Disease Research,* Geneva.
- WHO (2000). Roll Back Malaria : Country Updates. *WHO/CDS/RBM/ 2000.24.,* pp : 1-80.

Chapter - 6
Malaria : Clinical Features and Treatment

Asim Krishna De

Abstract

Malaria has been the enemy of man since the ancient times. Even though new methods of treatment and different management policies are been formulated, the disease still haunts the human being. In this article, the history, types of malarial parasites, clinical features, treatment and some methods of prevention are being discussed.

History

About 1.5 million years ago, man-ape a bigger brained creature named *Homoerectus* made crucial journey out of Africa to Asia, as there was land bridge between the two continents. In Asia Erectus man might have first become malarious. Southeast Asia was the : "home and birth place" of numerous species of primate malaria, some of which was analogous to parasites at present day and was capable of infecting humans. Two of those monkey malaria parasites became humanized. *Plasmodium cymmonolgi* became *Plasmodium vivax* (B) and *Plasmodium inui* became *Plasmodium malariae*, the parasite of Qurtan malaria.

It was in 1880 that Laveran, a French army surgeon described malaria parasite in red blood cells of human being. Manson - Bar in the year 1894 suggested that malaria parasites are carried by mosquito, and its cycle of development takes place in mosquito. Sir Ronald Ross confirmed it in 1897. In the year 1899 Grassi, Bignani discovered the complete developmental cycle of *P. falciparum, P. vivax* and *P. malariae* and the whole cycle of sporogony of all malaria parasites was detailed by Grassi in the year 1900.

---

* 35, Garpar Road, Kolkata-700 009

Malaria Parasites and their transmission

1847 Dempster in India introduced spleen palpation of children as an index of malaria.

1880 Laveran in Algeria discovered and described malaria parasites in human blood.

1886 Golgi in Italy described in details two species at human parasites (*P. vivax and P. malariae*)

1889-90 Celli and Marchiafava in Italy described *P. falciparum.*

1894 Manson put forward the theory that malaria is transmitted from person to person by mosquito.

1897 Ronald Ross - discovered pigmented cysts (oocysts) on stomach wall of an Anopheles mosquito in India.

1898 Grassi, Bignami in Italy described the cycle of human malaria parasites in Anopheles mosquito.

1931 James revived Grassi's theory suggested that the sporozoite, soon after entering the body invades reticulo-endothelial cells or cells lining the capillary blood vessels.

1950 Garnham described pre-erythrocytic forms of *P. inui,* a quartan like parasite.

Types of Malarial Parasite

There are four generally recognised species of malaria parasites of human and their colloquial names (which have now become obsolete) are:

1. *P. malariae* (Laveran 1881) Quartan
2. *P. vivax* (Grassi and Febth 1890) Benign tertian, Simple tertian.
3. *P. falciparum* Welch - 1897 MT (Malignant tertian).
4. *P. ovale Stephens* - 1922 Ovale tertian.

The life cycle of all species of human malaria parasites is same. It comprises an exogenous sexual phase (Sporogony) with multiplication in Anopheles mosquito and an endogenous asexual phase (Schizogony) with multiplication in the vertebrate host.

Stages of four species human parasites

Species	Duration of sporogony in Anopheles	Diameter of mature oocyst	Appearance of pigment in oocyst	Duration of mature preerythro-cytic schizonts	Mean diameter preeryth-rocytic schizonts
P.vivax	8-10 days	50 µm	Feathery	6-8 days	45 µm
P.malar-iae	14-16 days	40 µm	Clustered at periphery	14-16 days	55 µm
P.ovale	12-14 days	45 µm	Crossed lines	9 days	60 µm
P.falcipa-rum	9-10 days	55 µm	Rows and chain	5 ½ - 7 days	60 µm

Plasmodium malariae

P. malariae is called quartan because the paroxysms occur on 4th day after an interval of 2 days. Parasites differ from other species by its morphological character and its slow development in both the mosquito and man host.

No direct evidence of pre-erythrocytic stages of *P. malariae* in human host is available. The infection with *P. malariae* has a tendency to persist in the human host for many years, probably due to successive secondary exo- erythrocytic cycle in the liver. As hypnozoites responsible for relapse do not exit in *P. malariae,* so reappearance of clinical symptoms may be due to exacerbation of primary attack from erythrocytes persisting in internal organs.

Young trophozoites are not very different from *P. vivax.* The development of trophozoites takes about 54 hours. Schizonts divide into 8 merozoites. Merozoites occupy the entire erythrocytes and are arranged symmetrically around the centre and the term rosette is applied to Schizonts. The gametocytes develop in internal organs and appear in the peripheral blood when grown fully. Male gamete has a diffuse larger nucleus. The sporagonic cycle in the Anopheles takes 30-35 days at 20^{0}C. The pigments in oocyst are large brown granules and have a peripheral distribution.

Plasmodium vivax

This species of parasite occurs mostly in the temperate zones and large areas of tropics. Sporozoits of *P. vivax* differentiate after invading liver into early, primary tissue Schizonts or the hypnozoits. These hypnozoits are responsible for relapses of infection. The stimulus, which activates the latent hypnozoits and provoke relapse is unknown. During the erythrocytic development of *P. vivax* all blood forms are found in the circulation and most stages are larger than the other species. The young trophozoite or ring grows rapidly and exhibit the characteristic malaria pigment. Cytoplasmic pseudopodia is typical for this species. Large vacuole forms a hole in the ring until the division of nucleus occurs. Mature schizont has 12-18 merozoits. Merozoits invade fresh erythrocytes and entire cycle is repeated every 48 hours. It has a striking effect on red blood corpuscles (RBC), which gradually enlarges and becomes decolonised. A characteristic form of small reddish points appear and is known as Schuffner's dots. Gametocytes appear in the blood within 3 days. Both male and female are large, round or oval filling the whole host cell. Both micro and macro gametes contain numerous pigment granules. After shedding the flagela male fertilise female gametes. The sexual cycle takes 16 days at 20°C, and 8-10 days at 28°C. The young oocyst has a light brown pigment in the form of fine granules.

Plasmodium falciparum

P. falciparum is most highly pathogenic, so it is called malignant. A non-immune person unless treated properly terminates totally. The asexual development of *P. falciparum* in the liver involves only preerythrocytic phase and hypnozoits do not occur. The young ring forms of *P. falciparum* seen in peripheral blood are very small. In many of ring forms there may be two chromatin granules and marginal forms are fairly common. Several rings may be seen in the host cell. Rings with double chromatin dots and multiple infection of red cells are more common in *P. falciparum*. Presence of maturing or mature Schizonts of *P. falciparum* in the blood requires prompt treatment. Segmenting form of *P. falciparum* is recognized for having two solid grains of pigment.

The ring forms and older trophozoites usually disappear from the peripheral circulation after 24 hours but they are present in brain, heart, spleen intestine even bone marrow, where further development takes place. Segmenting forms of *P. falciparum* are recognized by two solid grains of pigment. In course of 24 hours parasites multiply by schizont. When schizont is fully grown it occupies 2/3rd of red cell. Finally it undergoes segmentation giving rise to 8 to 24 merozoites. Mature schizont is smaller than any other species but amount of parasites in the circulating blood is huge. Capillaries are blocked by clumps of infected RBC. which retains their normal size through all stages of development.

Gametocytes develop within inner organs but sometimes-young forms are seen in blood. They may be elongated spindle shaped or elliptic as they grow and lastly curved shape of mature gametocytes appear in the peripheral blood, and then undergone schizogony in 10 days. Body may be sausage shaped or crescentic. Female or macrogametocytes is more slender and longer than male. Nucleus is small and the pigment granules are closely aggregated round it. Number of gametocytes varies from 50,000 to 1,50,000 per μl of blood. Duration of sexual cycle of *P. falciparum* is 22 days at 20^{0}C. Pigment in oocyst is black and granules are relatively large. It forms a double circle around the periphery.

Plasmodium ovale

Plasmodium ovale produces similar type of fever like *P. Vivax*, but often with a prolonged latent period. The chance of relapse is lesser. The asexual erythrocytic cycle of *P. ovale* is similar to *P. Vivax* and extend over 48 hours. Schizonts contain about 15,000 merozoites, the nucleus is often enlarged. The young trophozoits measure about 1/3rd diameter of RBC. Schuffener's dots appear early and are more pronounced than *P. Vivax*. Schizonts may resemble those of *P. malariae*. They are rounded, compact and contain 8-10 nuclei, which are arranged around the periphery, surrounding the central clamp of pigment granules.

The gametocytes of *P. ovale* resemble those of *P. malariae* but the erythrocyte, which they invade, assumes the shape of oval. Female gametocytes have a small bluish nucleus. Male gametocyte when stained looks pale blue with redish tinge. Pigment of oocyst is dark brown and the granule forms chain in the centre of the cyst. Sporagony cycle in the mosquito takes 12-14 days at 28^{0}C for completion.

Clinical features of malaria

Malaria is a disease, which causes acute febrile illness with periodic febrile paroxysm occurring every 48 or 72 hours with an interval of a febrile symptoms and a tendency to relapse over months. The incubation period is the interval between infection and appearance of fever, or primary attack. The pre-patent period is the period from the time of infection to the discovery of malaria parasites in the blood. Predormal symptoms are malaise, fatigue and a desire to yawn and stretch the limbs, headache, pain in body, nausea, vomiting and slight fever.

Characteristics of infection with four species of human plasmodium

	P. vivax	*P. ovale*	*P. malaria*	*P. falciparum*
Preerythrocytic stage	6-8 days	9 days	14-16 days	5-7 days
Prepatent period	11-13 days	10-14 days	15-16 days	9-10 days
Incubation period	15 (12-17) or 6-12 months	(16-18) days	28 (18-40) days	12 (9-14) days
Erythrocytic cycle (hr)	48 hours	50 hours	72 hours	48 hours
Primary attack	Mild to moderate	Mild	Mild	Severe in nonimmune
Febrile paroxysm	8-12	8-12	8-10	16-30 or longer
Relapses	++	++	-	-
Period of recurrence	Variable	Variable	Very long	Short
Duration of untreated infection	1½-5 years	1½-5 years	3-50 years	1-2 years

There are about three stages found in malaria victims.

1. *Cold stage*

Feeling of cold followed by mild to violent shivering, chattering of teeth and shaking of whole body. Patient tries to cover himself and ask for more clothing. Skin is cold to touch but temperature is getting raised. Pulse is low and volume poor. Patient vomits, temperature shoots up and convulsion begins. This rigor lasts for 20-60 minutes then shivering ceases.

2. *Hot stage*

Patient feels warm and becomes hot, throws all his clothing. Headache becomes intense palpitation tachycardia, syncopial attack, nausea and vomiting increases. Temperature rises to 104-106^{0}C and patient becomes confused and delirious. Skin becomes dry, flushed. Pulse is full and bounding. This stage persists from 2 to 6 hours.

3. *Sweating stage*

Patient passes into sweating stage. Fever declines gradually and patient perspires profusely. Symptoms diminish and patient becomes exhausted and goes to sleep. Duration of typical attack is 8- 12 hours. Infection becomes severe when patient is left untreated and large number of schizontes rupture simultaneously. Interval of attack is 48 hours i.e. alternate day in *P. falciparum, P. vivax, P.*

ovale, but 72 hours in *P. malaria* (quartan) unless the parasites are eliminated by adequate treatment the attack is prolonged and infection depends on a balance between multiplication of parasites and counteraction of immuno response of the host.

Relapse of *P. vivax* and *P. ovale* result from reactivation of hypnozoits form of parasites in the liver. In *P. falciparum* and *P. malariae* occurs exacerbation of persistent undetectable parasitaemias in the absence of exo-erythrocytic cycle.

Falciparum malaria (malignant tertian)

It is responsible for more than 2 million yearly deaths all over the world. Partial immune people can tolerate its infection with trivial or no symptoms. But for non immune people it is a potential fatal disease. In falciparum infection illness starts with headache pain in body, nausea, vomitting mild diarrhoea and chill. There are intermittent chills and the fever is continuous or remittent as in enteric fever. Appearance of rash, *Herpes simplex* in lips, a tinge of jaundice, lymphadenopathy, hepatospleenomegaly makes the diagnosis difficult. In non immune cases disease can progress very rapidly and death may take place within 24 hours.

Cerebral malaria

This is the most notorious form of malaria. About 90 percent of patients become comatose before death from malaria. Usually there is a history of fever and non specific symptoms before impairment of consciousness or a generalised convulsion followed by coma. In high fever irritability, confusion, delirium, drowsiness is very common. The term encephalopathy in *P. falciparum* is issued when patient suffers from unrousable coma. Patient with open eye lie motionless or toss restlessly grinding teeth. Various involuntary movements are seen. Convulsions are generalised. There may be mild meningism, but no neck rigidity or photophobia. Dys conjugate gaze, convergent spasm nystagmus maybe present. Mouth is forcibly closed. Recovery occurs after 40 hours of coma and full consciousness ensures after 18 hours.

Cerebral malaria in children

Early symptoms include fever, irritability, and failure to feed convulsion, cough, vomiting, and diarrhoea. Convulsion is very common and is generalised. Unlike adults children show abnomalities of corneal, occular vestibular reflexes, but papillary reflexes are normal. Muscular hypotonia is more common. Most deaths occur within 24 hours. Hypertension is frequent. In survivors duration of coma is shorter, and after 30 hours patient regains full consciousness.

Other features of severe falciparum malaria

Anaemia - Children under 2 years and pregnant woman suffer more from anemia. Severity of anaemia is correlated with parasitaemia and schizontaemia. There may be retinal haemorrhage and kidney dysfunction. Exchange transfusion is a safe way of treating anaemia.

Jaundice and liver dysfunction

Jaundice is more common in adult. Liver and spleen are enlarged and tender. Liver failure and hepatic encephalopathy does not occur, unless there is concomittee viral hepatitis. But sometimes serum bilirubin and output of urobilirubinogen are increased, and jaundice is developed in severe cases.

Hypoglycaemia

Anxiety, feeling of coldness, tachycardia, impairment of consciousness, seizures - the classical symptoms of hypoglycaemia are likely to be found. In pregnant woman with severe or uncomplicated falciparum infection hypoglycaemia is common also in patients treated with quinine and quinidine. Intravenous glucose shows much improvement in hypoglycaemia and neurological malfunctions.

Renal dysfunction

This is another complication of falciparum infection. Most of non immune adult develops evidence of renal dysfunction with oliguria, or anuria.

Hyperpyrexia

Core (rectal) temperature should be monitored regularly and should not be allowed to rise above 39^{0}C, as the temperature is associated with clinical dehydration and febrile convulsion, delirium etc. Treatment includes water sponging all over the body, i.v. transfusion, cold rectal saline and drugs like paracetamol and nimuselide may be given to lower temperature.

Shock-algid malaria and cardiovascular abnormalities

It is characterized by collapse and coldness of extremities, and a tendency to fatal syncope. Although axillary and rectal temperature remains high blood pressure becomes at the lowest range. Gastrointestinal symptoms are associated with passage of blood and mucus present in the stool.

Pulmonary oedema

It is the most dangerous complication of malaria, it may be due to excessive parasitic fluid therapy. Early signs are increased respiratory rate, dyspnaea, etc. X-Ray will confirm diagnosis.

Chemotherapy and chemoprophylaxis of malaria

Antimalarial drugs have selective action on different phases of parasite life cycle. Prophylactic drugs prevent the establishment of parasite in liver.

(1) Schinzonticidal drugs - Which attack the parasite in R.B.C. preventing or terminating the clinical attack. Gametocytocidal drug destroy the sexual form of parasite in blood, some of these drug are hypnozoaitocidal (that will kill hypnozoites in liver and prevent relapse).

(2) Sporonticidal drugs - Inhibit the development of oocysts on the stomach wall of mosquito so that mosquito cannot transmit infection.

(3) Sporonticidal drugs - Proguanil, Pyrimethamine.

(4) Tissue schizontocidal drugs - Proguanil, Pyrimethamine, Pamaquin, Primaquin.

(5) Hypnozoitocidal drugs - Pamaquine, Primaquine.

(6) Gametocytocidal drugs - Pamaquin, Primaquin, Metakelfin, Fansidar.

(7) Blood Schizontocidal drugs - Chloroquine, Quinine, Quinidine, Amodiaquine, Maefloquin, Artimesin, Fansidar (Sulphadoxine 1500 mg + 75 mg pyrimethamine 3 lant a time) or Metakelfin.

Treatment and prevention of malaria

(I) Protective (prophylactive)

Absolute prevention of infection means destruction of sporozoits soon after they have been inoculated by the bite of a female Anopheles mosquito - There is no drug that can prevent it. There are drugs which act on parasites when it is within the liver tissue before merozoites are liberated into the blood. Schizonticidal drugs have little effect on liver, but if it is present in the blood when merozoites live in the liver and invade erythrocytes, this drug will definitely prevent malaria.

(II) Curative (therapeutic)

Schizonticidal drugs are used during active attack, in relapsing malaria and for radical treatment.

(III) Preventive

Drugs acts on gametocytes in peripheral blood of human host interrupting the stages of sporogonic phase in mosquito.

Quinine

This alkaloid of Cinchona has been in use for centuries. Quinine is still the treatment of choice in chloroquine resistant cases of falciparum infection. It is absorbed by the intestinal tract, and about 20 percent is excreted in the urine and the rest is passed to the liver where transformation takes place to hydroxyquinine and other metabolites. Plasma concentration reaches about 1-3 hour, and elimination time about 11-18 hours. It is most valuable in the treatment of severe falciparum infection. In Quinine after dilution 20 mg per kg body wt. can be infused over 4 hours. It can be given by intramuscular route into anterior part of thigh. Although possibility of muscle necrosis is there. Oral dose of quinine of 10 mg per kg of body wt. is given to adults. Rubiquin or Qinarsola 600 mg BD for 9-10 days or 600 mg TDS for 5 days may be given depending upon the condition and severity of infection. It is an schizonticidal drug and acts by interfering with the lysosomal function of parasites or nucleic acid synthesis of plasmodia. It has no action at the exo erythrocytic stage. Quinine in conventional doses has proved safe in pregnancy.

The toxic effects of quinine includes deafness, tenitus, nausea, vomiting, dizziness blurring of vision, malaise. Sometimes quinine may cause haemolysis, severe thrombocytopenia in coagulation, central nervous system and cardiovascular toxicity including blindness, coma, convulsion, hypotension myocardial conduction disturbance and severe toxic effects like hyperinsulinaemia, hypoglycemia etc.

Quinidine

It is more effective than quinine against *P. falciparum* but is more cardiotoxic.

Mefloquine

It is quinoline methanol similar to quinine and has a long lasting schizontcidal effect against all types of malaria including *P. falciparum* - resistant to aminoquinolene (chloroquine) - pyrimethamine - sulphonamide concentration and quinine. Given orally it is well absorbed, peak level 11-48 hours, elimination half life 6-33 days. In cerebral malaria mefloquin suspension is absorbed rapidly but bio - availability is reduced. Mefloquin can be given in single doses in adult and children (15-25 mg/kg body wt). To reduce gastrointestinal toxicity it can be given in two halves 6-8 hours apart. It is proved as first line of treatment in *P.falciparum* but usually it is used as second line of treatment and is associated with some toxic effects like - dizziness, nausea, vomiting, abdominal colic, sinus bradycardia, sinus arrhythmia and postural hypotension. An acute mid-brain syndrom-failure, sthenia seizures, psychos can also be seen. It can be used prophylactically (250 mg weekly)

Dose	Confal 250 mg -	5 tabs
	Mefloc 250 mg -	4 tabs
	Mefliam 250 mg -	6 tabs
Upto 60 kg	3 tabs stat -	2 tabs after 6-8 hours
Over 60 kg	3 tabs stat + 2 tabs after 6-8 hours + 1 tabs after 6-8 hours.	

Drug should not be taken in empty stomach but with atleast 250 ml. of water.

Chloroquine

It is the most widely used drug of malaria. It acts mostly in all the types of malaria parasites viz. *P. vivax, P. malariae, P. ovale* and also in *P. falciparum*. It is slightly effective against schizonts and even gametocytes stages of malaria parasites. Due to the extensive use of chloroquine, many resistant cases of *P.falciparum* or *P. vivax* have been found recently. It is absorbed rapidly and the peak plasma concertration reaches within 2 hours. The bioavailability is 70-75 %. As it is absorbed very quickly so, intra muscle or subcutaneous injections are given (2.5 to 3.5 mg/kg) 6 hourly maximum. intra venous - in *P. falciparum* 10 mg/kg infused over 8 hours followed by 15 mg/kg over 24 hours. The oral dose is 600 mg followed by 300 mg for 6-8 hours interval, 300 mg after 24 hours and 300 mg after 48 hours, if temperature persists again 300 mg after 72 hours.

As prophylaxis

300 mg or 250 mg weekly for 8 weeks; children 5 mg/kg

Toxic doses cause nausea, headache, drowsiness, malaisa, blurring of vision, speech, abnormalities, jaw contraction, involuntary moving of head, syncopial attack, hypokalamia, thrombocytopenia, respiratory paralysis, sometimes cardiac arrest, tachycardia, prolonged Qt. Diazepam and adrenaline counteracts the chloroquin on myocardium and blood vessel. Phenargan, because of its antiallergic and antiemetic effect is used with chloroquine and Domperidon. Ing. Of avil sometimes gives beneficial effects.

Mepacrine

It was introduced in the market in the year 1930 but after few years was discarded for its toxicity. It was found to be deposited in the skin causing yellow colour, yellow vision and mental disturbances. Sometimes it is used in treatment of giardiasis.

Amodiaquin (camoquin)

Its action is like chloroquine, but it is too much toxic. It causes toxic hepatitis, agranulocytosis etc and has been discarded.

Primaquine

Aminoquinoline is the only drug, which kills the hyponozoites of relapsing *P. vivax* and *P. ovale*. For this reason it is used for radical cure of *P. vivax* but as it causes haemolysis in patients with erythrocytes enzyme deficiencies (glucose-6-phosphate dehydrogenase) it should be given in caution. Doses -7.5 mg twice daily for 14 days after a course of chloroquine.

Tetracycline

It is an useful addition to quinine in chloroquinine resistant cases.

Amoxycillin

It is an effective drug for multiresistant falciparum and mefloquin resistant cases. Dose is 1000-2000 mg daily. It should not be given in pregnant and lactating women, and children under the age of 8 years as it has a damaging effect on development of bone and teeth.

Artemether

It is a Chinese preparation and is effective against chloroquine resistant, falciparum infections including cerebral malaria. It is a schozonticidal drug.

Dose - 1 amp BD on 1st day followed by 1 amp. O.D. (80 mg) for subsequent 4 days.

Larither Ing. 80 mg amp.

Cap 40 mg BD for one day then one daily for 4 days

Interacts with quinidine, amodiarone sotalal, astemezoli, phenothiazine, adverse reactions like nausea, vomiting, abdomonal pain, bradycardia; and first degree heart block.

Drugs which reverse chloroquine resistance

Chloroquine is excreted from parasites food vacuoles, so lethal concentration does not reach the cytoplasm. Ca-channel blocker e.g. (verapanil and nifidipine) Cyproheptadin Ketotifen, effectively reverse the resistance of chloroquine.

Treatment of uncomplicated malaria

Chloroquine is the treatment of choice of all types of malaria. But despite the clinical improvement following chloroquine treatment its failure to eradicate and subsequent recrudescence may develop severe anaemia, particularly in children. If anaemia is present chloroquine be replaced with Fansider or Croydoxon. Metattefin (Pyrimethamine-Sulfonamide combination) has great advantage of being single dose treatment. Short course of quinine followed by Pyrimethamen + Sulfonamide combination is still effective. Most antimalarial drugs taste bitter. So generous drink of milk, fruit juice or flavoured fluid can be given after taking antipyretic (Paracitamol) antimalarial drugs.

Black water fever

In certain cases of *P. falciparum* infection acute haemolysis occurs followed by haemoglobinaemia and haemoglobinuria. This type of syndrome is called Black Water Fever. It occurs in people exposed frequently in endemic areas of *P. falciparum*. Irregular attack of *P. falciparum* infection produce some kind of sensitivity reaction which response to further infection by acute intravascular haemolysis with fever, jaundice and renal insufficiency. This haemolysis leads to severe anaemia. Haemoglobinuria develops suddenly. Urine becomes dark brown or black. Its reaction may be acid, alkaline or neutral. Urine may contain dark brown pigment and protein. Its volume is low and anuria may develop. Death may occur from haemolysis, vascular collapse or acute hepatic failure or uramia.

Treatment

Corticosteroids in the early stages are helpful. Transfusion is necessary in case of Renal failure, Dehydration, Hepatic failure and Shock.

Endemic malaria

Manifestation of malaria in people grown up in the endemic area vary with the age of patient and the development of immunity. In hypoendemic areas little immunity is acquired , so the people affected by malaria do not differ from non-immune persons. In mesoendemic areas malaria is frequent but only seasonal. So frequent attacks of malaria lead to anaemia and enlargement of spleen to the extent of rupture. In hyperendemic areas, malaria occurs throughout the year and people develop considerable immunity.

Tropical splenomegaly syndrome

In hyperendemic areas splenomegaly is associated with exaggerated immune response to malaria. People particularly female who have high antibody titres to malaria and low parasitaemia, enormous over production of lgM levels reaching 3-20 times that of local mean value. Much of lgM is aggregated to other immunoglobulin. lgM aggregated are phagocytosed by reticuloendothelial cells in the spleen and liver.

Diagonsis

Malaria should be considered if a febrile patient has come from malarious locality. Acute febrile splenomegaly with anaemia may be a case of malaria. Well stained blood film (thick and thin) should be repeated if necessary to confirm the diagnosis. In partial or uncomplicated cases *P.falciparum* parasites are very scanty. Ring form is found in early cases; with other species all stages of erythrocytic cycle may be found.

Gametocytes appear after about 2 weeks. Malaria may coexist with other diseases and not because of illness in semi-immune persons in endemic areas.

Principles of malaria prevention and control

1. Measures be taken to prevent mosquito from biting human.
2. Measures be designed to prevent breeding of mosquito by draining the collection of water and improve the condition of environment.
3. Measures be designed to destroy the larvae of mosquitoes.
4. Measures be taken to destroy adult mosquito.
5. Measures be taken to eliminate the malaria parasite in human host.

Protection against mosquito

Nets: It is the easiest and most convenient way of preventing mosquito bites at night and has been practiced from a very early time. Nylon nets are light and easy to carry. If the nets are impregnated with the solution of permethrin, (which is also a mosquito repellent) very good results are found.

Protective clothing: It also includes covering of hands and feets using thick socks and hand gloves. In forest areas sleeves should be rolled down after sunset, morning and even in daytime.

Mosquito repellents: These are substances applied to the skin, clothing or nets to repel mosquitoes and prevent them from biting. The drugs used are (i) Dimethylphthlate DBP - Dibutylphthalate. Their average protection are 3-4 hours but DEET appears to be best and its action is 10 hours. It should be applied liberally over the neck, ankles and wrists (face, eyelids are to be avoided). Mosquito coils, mats or joss sticks containing Pyrethrum are useful as a type of repellent. Smoke from coils/ joss sticks are irritant to some and are to be avoided in case of children.

Screening: Doorframe fitted to strong wire nets and door open outwards, having a strong spring to ensure tight closing is good method of preventing mosquito entering in the room. It is an advantage to have double door, with a porch of atleast 2 m in length between them.

Mosquito control: Mosquito control is the best method of protecting humanity against malaria and other mosquito borne diseases. Source reduction is a very important method of mosquito control. Prevention of mosquito breeding in places like marshy land, unclean ditches, open drains, toilet, half constructed buildings, open cisterns, dumped sewage, dustbins, etc. should be routinely checked.

Moreover, the rising problem of resistance of mosquitoes to insecticides in public health programmes and in intensive agriculture, together with growing concern for the environment exposed to repeated application of toxic compounds is a matter of potential interest and is very difficult to solve. The need of the hour is to involve general public in fighting the menace of malaria bearing mosquitoes.

Reference

- Boland M. E. Brenaard Roper S. M. Henry J.A. (1985) Complication of Quinine Posioning *Lancet* 1384-5.
- Bray R.S. Granham P.C.C. (1982) Life cycle of malaria parasite *British Medical Bulletin* 38. 117-22.

- Davidson's. Principal and Practice of Medicine pp. 154.
- D. A. Warrel (1987) Malaria. In Oxford Textbook of Medicine 2nd Edition. pp. S.474-S. 502 Oxford University Press.

Chapter - 7
Artemisinin : The Drug for Malaria

**Amit Krishna De*

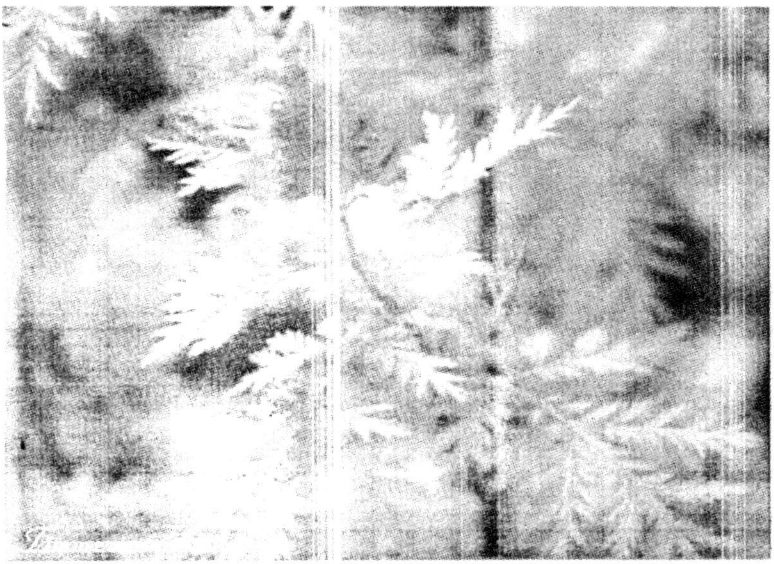

Sweet Annie (*Artemisia annua*) :

Abstract

Artemisia annua L., Asteraceae, a species native to China but naturalized in the United States, is the source of artemisinin (qinghaosu),

* Indian Science Congress Association, 14, Biresh Guha Street, Kolkata-700 017

an endoperoxide sesquiterpene lactone which is effective against sensitive and multi-drug resistant strains of Plasmodium, the malarial parasite.

Introduction

Artemisia (*Artemisia annua* L., Asteraceae), known in the United States as sweet Annie or annual wormwood, is an annual herb native to Asia, most probably China, where it is known as *qinghao.* The plant has become naturalized in many countries including Argentina, Bulgaria, France, Hungary, Romania, Italy, Spain, the United States, and the former Yugoslavia (Klayman 1989, 1993).

Botany

Artemisia annua, a vigorous weedy annual (Hall and Clements 1923), is a short day plant with a critical photoperiod of 13.5 hr (Ferriera *et al.* 1995a). The chromosome number is $2n = 36$ (Bennette *et al.* 1982). The plant is usually single-stemmed reaching about 2m in height with alternate branches and alternate, deeply dissected, aromatic leaves ranging from 2.5 to 5.0 cm in length. Tiny yellow nodding flowers (capitula) only 2 or 3 mm across are displayed in lose panicles containing numerous, greenish or yellowish, bisexual central (disc) florets containing little nectar and pistillate marginal (ray) florets. The involucre is imbricated with several rows and bracts. The central flowers are perfect and can be either fertile or sterile. Ovaries are inferior and unilocular and each generates one achene, ca. 1 mm in length and fainty nerved. The pistillate marginal florets in the capitulum produce numerous achenes without pappus. The pollen is tricolpate and smooth, typical of anemophilous species, and has vestigial or no spines (Stix 1960). It has an internal, complex, columellae-tecta configuration in the exine, which is common to all taxa of the tribe Anthemideae and varies from two to three layers in *A. annua* (Skvarla and Larson 1965). The plant is naturally cross-pollinated by insects and wind action, which is unusual in the Asteraceae (McVaugh 1984).

Non-glandular T-shaped trichomes and 10-celled biseriate glandular trichomes occur on leaves, stems, and inflorescences. The morphology and origin of the glandular trichomes has been described for leaves (Duke and Paul 1993) and capitula (Ferreira and Janick 1995) using light and/or scanning electron microscopy.

Constituents

The main active principle, artemisinin (formerly referred to as arteannuin and as *qinghaosu* in Chinese), was isolated and had its structure correctly defined in 1972 in China as a sesquiterpene lactone with an endoperoxide bridge. The essential oil of *A. annua* contains at least 40 volatile compounds and several nonvolatile sesquiterpenes, of which artemisinin and related compounds are the ones of most interest due to their antimalarial properties (Charles *et al.* 1991; Woerdenbag *et al.* 1994; Klayman, 1989, 1993).

Artemisinin is now available commercially in China and Vietnam as an antimalarial drug efficacious against drug-resistant strains of *Plasmodium*, the malarial parasite. A semisynthetic drug based on artemisinin (artemether) has been recently registered in Africa as Paluther. Artemisinin also has phytotoxic activity, even on *A. annua*, and is a candidate as a natural herbicide (Duke *et al.* 1987; *et al.* 1991).

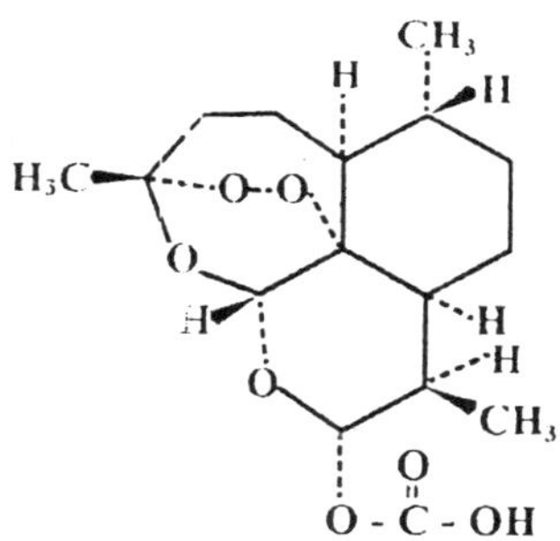

Artemisinin $C_{15}H_{24}O_5$

Artemisinin production by *A. annua* is usually in the range of 0.001% to 0.4% but some clones produce over 1% (Delabays *et al.* 1993). Artemisinin can also be obtained from artemisinic acid which occurs at concentration as much as 10-fold higher than artemisinin (Acton *et al.* 1985). Recently, Vonwiller *et al.* (1993) reported an extraction method which makes possible the extraction of both compounds from the same plant material, thus increasing the final production of artemisinin.

Artemisinin distribution

In vivo

Artemisinin can be quantified by various analytical procedures including thin layer chromatography, gas chromatography, high-performance liquid chromatography with ultraviolet or electrochemical detection (Ferreira *et al.* 1994), radioimmunoassay, and enzyme-linked immunosorbant assay (Ferreira and Janick 1996a). Artemisinin has been detected from aerial parts of the plant, mostly in leaves and inflorescences with low levels in stems and none in pollen or roots. The occurrence of artemisinin in the achene (seed) is due to the presence of floral remnants.

Some authors had reported artemisinin to be highest during preflowering stages (Acton *et al.* 1985; Liersch *et al.* 1986; Woerdenbag *et al.* 1991; El-Sohly 1990; Woerdenbag *et al.* 1994), others reported artemisinin reaching its peak during flowering Singh *et al.* 1988; Pras *et al.* 1991; Morales *et al.* 1993; Ferreira *et al.* 1995a; Laughlin 1995). Artemisinin reached its peak during full flowering in a Chinese clone for both greenhouse and field conditions (Ferreira *et al.* 1995b).

Reports on the distribution of artemisinin throughout the plant have been inconsistent. Artemisinin has been reported to be higher at the top of the plant in some clones (Charles *et al.* 1990; Laughlin 1995) and equally distributed in others (Laughlin 1995). Six clones derived from Chinese material were analyzed during both vegetative and flowering stages with samples taken from the bottom, middle, and top parts of the plant, and a relatively even distribution of artemisinin was found along the main stem. Five of the six clones showed the same or higher levels of artemisinin at the flowering stage. Although plants from all clones were harvested at the same date, they were in different stages of development. Branches of one clone were collected sequentially from the bottom to the top of the plant. In this clone artemisinin showed a slight increase in artemisinin toward the top of the plant.

In vitro

Artemisinin is produced by differentiated (shoots + roots) shoot cultures (Martinez and Staba 1988; Fulzele *et al.* 1991; Whipkey *et al.* 1992; Ferreira and Janick 1996b) but occurs only in trace levels, if at all, in shoots without roots (Jha *et al.* 1988; Woerdenbag *et al.* 1993; Paniego and Giuliette 1994). Brown (1994) reported 0.0038% of artemisinin being produced by callus cultures bearing shoots but did not specify whether or not they had roots. Most workers (Martinez and Staba 1988; Tawfiq *et al.* 1989; Fulzele *et al.* 1991; Kim *et al.* 1992) did not detect artemisinin in roots, although Nair *et al.* (1986) and Jha *et al.* (1988) reported trace amounts. Weathers *et al.* (1994) reported high levels (0.4%) of artemisinin in hairy root cultures of *A. annua* transformed with *Agrobacterium rhyzogenes*, but this was not confirmed by Jaziri *et al.* (1995). With the exception of Jha *et al.* (1988),most authors (He *et al.* 1983; Nair *et al.* 1986;

Tawfiq *et al.* 1989; Fulzele *et al.* 1991; Kim *et al.* 1992; Woerdenbag *et al.* 1993; Brown 1994; Paniego and Giuliette 1994; Ferreira and Janick 1996b) either reported to artemisinin or only trace amounts produced from callus, cell, or the spent liquid media from these cultures. Ferreira and Janick (1996b) presented evidence that artemisinin production in shoots was enhanced by the presence of roots. The highest levels of artemisinin (0.287% DW) were obtained in hormone-free medium when the root production was maximized.

Glandular trichomes as sites of artemisinin accumulation

Although artemisinin immunolocalization has not been achieved, there is strong circumstantial evidence that the compound is sequestered in the glandular trichomes. Duke and Paul (1993) and Duke *et al.* (1994) described the development of such glands in leaves of *A. annua* and reported that neither artemisinin or artemisitene were detected from a glandless biotype and that virtually all artemisinin could be extracted by a 5-sec leaf dip in chloroform, without visible damage to other leaf epidermal cells, from the biotype with glands.

Artemisinin content (%DW) was shown to be 4 to 11 times higher in the inflorescences as compared to leaves (Ferreira *et al.* 1995a) and the presence and development of glandular trichomes in the inflorescences was associated with artemisinin production based on extraction studies (Ferreira and Janick 1995). The glandular trichomes are more prominent in the corolla and receptacles florets than in leaves, stems, or bracts. Although these glands are present since the early stage of development on both leaves and inflorescences, artemisinin increases at anthesis, suggesting that it accumulates as the glands reach physiological maturity, a stage which coincides with the end of cell expansion in floret development. As glands approach maturity, there appears to be a cellular discharge into the subcuticular space around the apical cells and contents are spread over the epidermis when the glands burst. After anthesis, artemisinin decreases and so does the number of intact glands. The association of artemisinin with glandular trichomes sequestration explains why artemisinin was not detected in parts of the plant that do not bear glands, such as pollen or roots (Ferreira *et al.* 1995a) or in a glandless biotype (Duke *et al.* 1994). Glandular trichomes are observed in leaves and stems of differentiated shoot cultures and artemisinin content of shoot cultures *in vitro* was similar to artemisinin content in vegetative clones grown in the greenhouse (Ferreira *et al.* 1995b).

Historical or traditional uses

Ancient Chinese medical texts dating from around 150 B.C. suggest the use of sweet Annie for people with hemorrhoids (Foster *et al.* 1992). Other writing from 340 A.D. are the first known to mention sweet Annie as a treatment for people with fevers. It has been used ever since for a variety of infections in traditional Chinese medicine. Artemisia is mentioned in the *Chinese Handbook of Prescriptions for Emergency Treatments* of 340 AD for treatment of fevers. In 1971, extraction of aerial parts of *A. annua* with lowboiling solvents, such as diethylether, produced a compound mixture with antimalarial properties on infected mice and monkeys.

Antimalarial actions

Artemisinin is believed to cause free radical damage to the red blood cells of the organism that infects. Artemesinin kills the sythrocytic stage of the sexual reproduction cycle of *Plasmodium*. Numerous un-blinded but randomized clinical studies, and some double-blind ones, have shown that injections or oral amounts of artemisinin or similar compounds rapidly and effectively cure people with malaria. Randomized, open, clinical studies have shown that artemisinin reduced mortality due to malaria by 50% compared with treatment with a standard quinoline anti-malarial drug. Artemisinin based drugs have not been studied for prevention of malaria. Test tube studies suggest artemisinin can kill other parasites and bacteria (Bone *et al.*, 1992), supporting the traditional notion of using it for parasitic infections of the gastrointestinal tract. Artemesinin is indicated for the treatment of malaria caused by all forms of *Plasmodium* including uncomplicated and severe complicated malaria. It is effective against malaria caused by chloroquine resistant strains of *Plasmodium falciparum*. It is also suitable for the treatment of pernicious malaria. Doctor often use sweet Annie in combination with other anti-parasitic herbs.

The antimalarial drug artemisinin is the weapon of choice for the treatment of cerebral malaria caused by the protozoon *Plasmodium falciparum*. But the drug can only be produced in small quantities. Researchers at the Jawaharlal Nehru Technology University in Hyderabad (*Biochem. Biophys, Commun* 281,2001) reports that Artemisinin is produced by the enzymatic conversion of the intermediate precursor anteannuin-B. Endogenous production of artemisinin is just 0.05% to 1.1%, however, which pushes up the price of the drug. Chemical synthesis of artemisinin is complex and uneconomical. Researchers have found a way of raising the yield of artemisinin from the plant. They have successfully isolated the enzyme involved in the conversation of arteannun-B to artemisinin in the plant's leaves and have purified and characterized it. The pure protein, which has a relative molecular mass of 66,000 is most active at a temperature of 30^{0}C. Biotransformation of arteannuin-B (extracted from the plant leaves) into artemisinin can now be done in a reactor using this pure enzyme and some cofactors. According to the researchers there are two reasons for the increased yield of artemisinin. First, levels of arteannuin-B, are about three times higher that of artemisinin during certain stages of plant growth, so there is more of the precursor to start with. The second reason is that the purified enzyme has been shown to convert 58% of arteannuin-B into artemisinin in laboratory experiments. This is the first time that this enzyme has been isolated and purified. The additional advantage is that the enzyme can be immobilized in calcium alginate beads. The enzyme remained active for three operational cycles, indicating that its use could be optimized by immobilization for industrial applications. The new *in vitro* biotransformation process, if it is combined with tissue culture cultivation of the plant, could potentially bring down the cost of artemisinin. The scientists are now looking for an industrial partner to help them scale up the process.

Conclusion

Artemisinin is a sesquiterpene lactone which is produced both *in vivo* and differentiated *in vitro* cultures, by *Artemisia annua* and is equally distributed throughout the plant. Artemisinin appears to be sequestered in glandular trichomes which occur in stems, leaves, and inflorescences. The association of peak artemisinin with flowering is related to the abundance of glandular trichomes in the inflorescence, particularly florets and receptacle. *In vitro* studies indicate that the biosynthesis of artemisinin is enhanced by the presence of roots. *Artemisia annua* is unlikely to be produced economically by chemical synthesis or by *in vitro* production, thus *A. annua* is a potential new antimalarial crop for temperate areas.

References

- Acton, N., D. L. Klayman, and I. J. Rollman. (1985). Reductive electrochemical HPLC assay for artemisinin (qinghaosu). *Planta Med.* **51** : 445-446.

- Bailey, L. H. and E. Z. Bailey. (1976). *Hortus third.* MacMillan Publ. Co., New York.
- Bennett, M. D., J. B. Smith, and J. S. Heslop-Harrison. (1982). Nuclear DNA amounts in angiosperms. *Proc. Royal Soc. London* **B 216** : 179-199.
- Brown, G. D. (1994). Secondary metabolism in tissue culture of *Artemisia annua. J. Nat. Prod.* **57(7)** : 975-977.
- Bone K, Morgan M. (1992) *Clinical Applications of Ayurvedic and Chinese Herbs : Monographs for the Western Herbal Practitioner.* Warwick, Australia : Phytotherapy Press, 7-12.
- Charles, D.J., E.Cebert, and J.E. Simon.(1991). Characterization of the essential oils of *Artemisia annua L. J. Ess. Oil Res.* **3** : 33-39.
- Charles, D.J., J.E. Simon, K.V. Wood, and P. Heinstein (1990). Germplasm variation in artemisinin content of *Artemisia annua* using an alternative method of artemisinin analysis from crude plant extracts. *J. Nat. Prod.* **53** : 157-160.
- Chen, P.K., G. Leather, and M. Polatnick. (1991). Comparative study on artemisinin, 2, 4-D, and glyphosate. *J. Agr. Food Chem.* **39** : 991-994.
- Delabays, N., A. Benakis, and G. Collet. (1993). Selection and breeding for high artemisinin (qinghaosu) yielding strains of *Artemsia annua. Acta Hort.* **330**:203-206.
- Duke, S.O., K.C. Vaughn, E.M. Croom Jr., and H.N. Elsohly. (1987). Artemisinin, a constituent of annual wormwood *(Artemisia annua),* is a selective phytotoxin. *Weed Sci.* **35**:499-505.
- Duke, S.O. and R.N. Paul. (1993). Development and fine structure of glandular trichomes of *Artemisia annua L. Int. J. Plant Sci.* **154(1)**: 107-118.
- Duke, M.V., R.N. Paul, H.N. Elsohly, G. Sturtz, and S.O. Duke. (1994). Localization of artemisinin and artemisitene in foliar tissues of glanded and glandless biotypes of *Artemisia annua L. Int. J. Plant Sci.* **155**:365-372.
- El-Sohly, H. N. (1990). A large scale extraction technique of artemisinin from *Artemisia annua. J. Nat. Prod.* **53**:1560-1564.
- Ferreira, J.F.S., D.J. Charles, K. Wood, J.E. Simon, and J. Janick. (1994). A comparison of gas chromatography and high performance liquid chromatography for artemisinin analyses. *Phytochem. Anal.* **5**:116-120.
- Ferreira, J.F.S., J. Janick. (1995). Floral morphology of *Artemisia annua* with special reference to trichomes. *Int. J. Plant Sci.* **156**:807-815.
- Ferreira, J.F.S., J. Janick. (1996a). Immunoquantitative analysis of artemisinin from *Artemisia annua* using polyclonal antibodies. *Phytochemistry* **41**:97-104.
- Ferreira, J.F.S., J. Janick. (1996b). Roots as an enhanching factor for the production of artemisinin in shoot cultures of *Artemisia annua. Plant Cell Tissue Organ Cult.* **44**:211-217.

- Ferreira, J.F.S., J. E. Simon, and J. Janick. (1995a). Developmental studies of *Artemisia annua*: Flowering and artemisinin production under greenhouse and field conditions, *Planta Med.* **61**:167-170.
- Ferreira, J.F.S., J. E. Simon, and J. Janick. (1995b). Relationship of artemisinin content of tissue-cultured, greenhouse-grown, and field-grown plants of *Artemisia annua. Planta Med.* **61**:351-355.
- Fulzele, D.P., A.T. Sipahimalani, and M.R. Heble. (19910. Tissue cultures of *Artemisia annua* : organogenesis and artemisinin production. *Phytother. Res.* **5**:149-153.
- Foster S, Yue CX. (1992) *Herbal Emissaries : Bringing Chinese Herbs to the West.* Rochester, VT: Healing Arts Press, 322.
- Hall, H.M. and F.E. Clements. (1923). The phylogenetic method in taxonomy. The North American species of *Artemisia, Chrysothamnus* and *Atriplex.* Carnegie Inst. Wash., Washington.
- He, X-C., M-Y. Zeng, G-F. Li, and Z. Liang. (1983). Callus induction and regeneration of plantlets from *Artemisia annua* and changes of qinghaosu contents. *Acta. Bot. son.* **25**:87-90.
- Jaziri, M., K. Shimomura, K. Yoshimatsu, M.-L. Fauconnier, M. Marlier, and J. Homes. (19950. Establishment of normal and transformed root cultures of *Artemisia annua* L. for artemisinin production. *J. Plant Physiol.* **145**:175-177.
- Jha, J., T.B. Jha, and S.B. Mahato. (1988). Tissue culture of *Artemisia annua* L.: A potential source of an antimalarial drug. *Curr. Sci.* **57**:344-346.
- Kim, N-C., J-G. Kim, H-J. Lim, T-R. Hahn, and S-U. Kim. (1992). Production of secondary metabolites by tissue culture of *Artemisia annua L. J. Korean Agr. Chem. Soc.* **35**:99-105.
- Klayman, D.L. (1989). *Weeding out malaria.* Nat. Hist. Oct.: 18-26.
- Klayman, D.L. (1993) *Artemisia annua* : From weed to respectable antimalarial plant. pp. 242-255. In: A. D. Kinghorn and M.F. Balandrin (eds.), Human Medicinal Agents from Plants. Am. Chem. Soc. Symp. Series. Washington, DC.
- Laughlin, J.C. (1995). The influence of distribution of antimalarial constituents in *Artemisia annua* L. on time and method of harvest. *Acta Hort.* **390**:67-73.
- Liersch, R., H. Soicke, C. Stehr, and H-U. Tullner. (1986). Formation of artemisinin in *Artemisia annua* during one vegetation period. *Planta Med.* **52**:387-390.
- Martinez, B.C. and J. Staba. (1988). The production of artemisinin in *Artemisia annua* L. tissue cultures. *Adv. Cell Cult.* **6**:69-87.
- McVaugh, R. (1984). Compositae. Vol. 12. Flora Novo-Galiciana: a descriptive account of the vascular plants of Western Mexico, ed. W.R. Anderson. University of Michigan Press, Ann Arbor.
- Morales, M.R., D.J. Charles, and J.E. Simon. (1993). Seasonal accumulation of artemisinin in *Artemisia annua* L. *Acta Hort.* **344**:416-420.

- Nair, M.S.R., N. Acton, D.L. Klayman, K. Kendrick, D.V. Basile, and S. Mante. (1986). Production of artemisinin in tissue cultures of *Artemisia annua. J. Nat. Prod.* **49**:504-507.
- Paniego, N.B. and A.M. Giuliette. (1994). *Artemisia annua* L.: dedifferentiated and differentiated cultures. *Plant Cell Tiss. Organ Cult.* **36**:163-168.
- Pras, N., J.F. Visser, S. Batterman, H.J. Woerdenbag, T.M Malingre, and C.B. Lugt. (1991). Laboratory selection of *Artemisia annua* L. for high artemisinin yielding types. *Phytochem. Anal.* **2**:80-83.
- Singh, A., R.A. Vishwakarma, and A. Husain. (1988). Evolution of *Artemisia annua* strains for higher artemisinin production. *Planta Med.* **54**:475-476.
- Skvarla, J.J. and D. A. Larson. (1965). An electron microscopy study of pollen morphology in the Compositae with special reference to the Ambrosiinae. *Grana Palinol.* **6**:210-269.
- Stix, E. (1960). Pollenmorophologische untersuchungen an Compositen. *Grana Palynol.* **2**:41-104.
- Tawfiq, N.K., L.A. Anderson, M.F. Roberts, J.D. Phillipson, D.H. Bray, and D.C. Warhurst. (1989). Antiplasmodial activity of *Artemisia annua* plant cell cultures. *Plant Cell Rep.* **8**: 425-428.
- Vonwiller, S.C., R.K. Haynes, G. King, and H.J. Wang. (1993). An improved method for the isolation of qinghao (artemisinic) acid from *Artemisia annua, Planta Med. Lett.* **59**:562-563.
- Weathers, P.J., R.D. Cheetham, E. Follansbee, and K. Tesh. (1994). Artemisinin production by transformed roots of *Artemisia annua. Biotech. Lett.* **16**:1281-1286.
- Whipkey, A., J.E. Simon, D.J. Charles, and J. Janick. (1992). In vitro production of artemisinin from *Artemisia annua L. J. Herbs Spices Med. Plants.* **1**:15-25.
- Woerdenbag, H.J., N. Pras, R. Bos, J.F. Visser, H. Hendriks, T.M. Malingre. (1991). Analysis of artemisinin and related sesquiterpenoids from *Artemisia annua* L. by combined gas chromatography/mass spectrometry. *Phytochem. Anal.* **2**:215-219.
- Woerdenbag, H.J., J.F.J. Luers, W. Van Uden, N. Pras, T.M. Malingre, and A.W. Alfermann. (1993). Production of the new antimalarial drug artemisinin in shoot cultures of *Artemisia annua L. Plant Cell Tiss. Organ Cult.* **32**:247-257.
- Woerdenbag, H.J., N. Pras, N.G. Chan, B.T. Bang, R. Bos, W van Uden, P. van Y., N.V. Boi, S. Batterman, and C.B. Lugt. (1994). Artemisinin, related sesquiterpenes, and essential oil in *Artemisia annua* during a vegetation period in Vietnam. *Planta Med.* **60**:272-75.

Chapter - 8

Quality Assurance in Diagnostic, Therapeutic and Control Measures in Malaria

A.K. Hati[1], B. Mondal[2], N.K. Mitra[3], H. Mukherjee[4], A. Mukhopadhyay[5] and S. Sengupta[6]

Abstract

Malaria is one of the most puzzling infectious diseases with a serious public health threat. This has been accentuated because quality assurance is not maintained or adhered to in diagnostic, therapeautic and control procedures. As a result a great deal of confusion exists in these fields, though there are standard literature and methods which are not so difficult to follow. But as the issue is very sensitive, everybody wants to be a self-styled authority setting aside, barring, ignoring or violating the established norms. The purpose of this paper is to point out that quality assurance can be instituted for the benefit of diagnosis, treatment and control of malaria.

Quality assurance in diagnosis

(i) Both thick and thin films are to be examined. Thin film is preferably stained with Leishman, thick film with Giemsa. For staining with Giemsa, standard W.H.O. technique is to be followed. A 10% Giemsa solution i.e. 3 drops of Giemsa per ml of buffer water solution having pH 7.1 is required. Blood

---

1. USERA, Science & Techonology, Govt. of India and Ex-Director STM, Kolkata-700073
2. Pathologist, ESI Hospital, Kolkata- 700009
3. Chief Pathologist, Gautam Laboratories, Kolkata-700007
4. M.O. Dept. of Medical Entomology, Kolkata-700003
5. Dy. Director, NMEP, Regional office for Health and Family Welfare, Kolkata- 700029
6. Director, CNCHS, Kolkata- 700031

film is stained for 5 minutes then the slide is washed gently in tap water, drained, dried and examined. In out laboratory, success rate to detect parasite is 28% more in thick films than in thin films. But even when thick films are negative, thin films may be positive, as possibility of washing out the parasite is there in the thick films. Secondly the thin film is more valuable for identifying the species of parasite present. However, if the parasite density is very low, it is diffcult or impossible to find any in the thin film.

(ii) Searching field in the thick film is it be 200 before declaring it negative. It takes about 5 minutes.

(iii) If only thin film is obtained, at least 15 minutes should be spent to examine before declaring it negative.

(iv) Number of slides a technician is to examine is 60/days.

(v) Counting of parasite capery little importance is given to count the parasite which can provide a lot of information:

Firstly, the density of *P. falciparum* is often related to severe malaria,

Secondly, evaluation of a drug, whether the parasite has become resistant to the drug used,

Thirdly parasite clearance time,

Fourthly, the degree of resistance can be adjudged if parasitaemia is counted on day 0, 3, 7 and 14.

For counting, one practical method in thin film is to find out number of rings of *P. falciparum*/1000 RBCs and at least 10,000 RBCs are to be scanned. If the count is 5/100 RBC, the condition is said to be serious. The second method is to count parasites in the thick fields per 200 leucocytes employing the formula.

$$\frac{\text{No. of parasites}}{\text{No. of leucocytes}} \text{ X } 8000 = \text{parasites/ml of the blood}$$

If the number of parasite is 100,000/ml, the patient is considered to be serious.

(vi) Time to take blood smear. There is a general belief that malaria blood is to be taken when there is fever. The idea is erroneous, chance to get parasite is more at the afebrile stage. For practical purposes, the slide should be taken at any time, when the fever is present or when the patient is in afebrile period.

(vii) How many times the blood should be taken? It depends on the condition of the patient, may be at the interval of 4, 6, 12 or 24 hours to detect malaria, where only blood slide examination facility is present.

(viii) Detection of antigen (HRP11). This is a new commercially available technique for detetion of *P. falciparum* antigen. Such test is also available against *P. vivax*. This test can be done within minutes without any other laboratory facility and even without electricity. The specificity and sensitivity are very high. But the facility is being misutilized. If the slide becomes negative and there is still a clinical suspicion, the test is justified. Another justification is to ascertain the species of parasite, when any confusion exists even after examination of the slide. In our laboratory 1000 tests to detect *P. falciparum* specific antigen showed the following results : antigen positive, but slide negative in 14 (1.4%) cases, antigen negative but slide positive in 3 (0.3%) cases. This test cannot quantify parasitaemia and may remain positive even after parasites disappear from the blood as a result of successful treatment, hence not suitable to evaluate drug resistance. This test is helpful in doubtful and severe cases. If stored in the ordinary refrigerator the antigen may remain for many years.

Quality assurance in the treatment

(i) *Fever clearance time* can easily be noted but no data is existing. In our study it was found to be 7-48 h, 24-48 h, 8-48 h and 0-48 h when treated with chloroquine, sulphadoxineaw and pyrimethamine, quinine and artemether respectively. It may be stressed that fever clearance time is not exactly related to drug sensitiveness or resistance. For example, both in chloroquine sensitive and grade 1 resistant cases fever may disappear after about 10 hours of taking first dose or may even persist for 48 hours. But persistence of fever for 3-4 days and aggravation of symptoms and / or appearance of complications should raise the suspicion of drug resistance.

(ii) *Parasite clearance time* is also not practised, which is immensely important in the present situation to evaluate degree of resistance. Clinical and parasitological response on day 3 and days 4-14 can be used as clear examples of early and late treatment failure. In a present series in 15 chloroquine resistant falciparum cases, parasites persisted or appeared in the blood with in 14 days in 9 cases and within 28 days in another 6 cases.

(iii) *Drug resistant falciparum cases.* In a high endemic area in Calcutta in a small series of cases (25) the pattern of drug sensitivity and resistance was as follows:

Chloroquine sensitive 12%, chloroquine resistant 40%, choloroquine resistant, but S & P sensitive 24%, S & P resistant 24%. This is a very small and biased sample but the indication is not at all good omen for the future.

In this scenario the treatment of falciparum malaria is becoming increasingly difficult as time is a very important factor. In low grade resistance, where recrudescence occurs between 7 and 28 days apparent cure, time to select drug and treat patient may be there, but in high grade (RII and RIII) resistance, where symptoms are aggravating and complications are appearing, the delay may be dangerous.

It seems that chloroquine may soon loose its position as the first choice of drug. S & P is also not so much reliable. Evaluation between quinine and tetracycline and artemesinin group of drugs is urgently needed so far as efficacy, tolerance, drug resistance and cost effectiveness are concerned.

(iv) *Use of primaquine.* Though primaquine is included in the national programme to kill the hyprnozoites of *P. Vivax* to prevent relapse, its use for that purpose in endemic area is practically useless as it cannot be possible to determine between a reinfection and a relapse. However, for falciparum malaria to kill gametocytes a stat dose of 45 mg is very much justified and for that G6PD examination is not essential according to W.H.O. Incidentally in a recent survey in our community G6PD deficient subjects were found to be about 3%.

Quality assurance in control

(i) Active case detection is one important pivot to control malaria. It is not existing. Hence malaria is spreading. Active case detection means regular home visit in search of fever cases and if fever cases are found, blood is taken and presumptive treatment is given.

As this is not being practised, patients are increasing in the community to transmit the disease. The problem is enormous. In 13454 falciparum cases, 1107 (8.2%) were found to possess gametocytes in the blood. In vivax malaria the corresponding figures were 21249 and 12080 (56.9%) respectively. They are actually the reservoirs, posing danger to the society. If active case detection is possible and presumptive treatment is given early, gametocyte circulation *vis a vis* spread of malaria in the community would be minimized.

(ii) *Source reduction of mosquito larvae.* This is another important pivot specially in the city of Calcutta. Source reduction is utterly and bitterly neglected.

(a) Each and every home is to be inspected for any source of breeding of mosquito and to be destroyed. This can be done by Govt. people, public health workers, corporation personnels, NGOs and general public.

(b) Ecofriendly modern biolarvicides can effectively kill the larvae in certain simation. This is to be enforced setting aside apathy and beurocracy barring its use.

(c) Fish, such as guppy etc can be released in the masonry tanks, which are main breeding sources. People should be motivated in that direction.

(iii) *Adulticid.* Foggins , mats, coils etc are not effective and the money is wasted. There is absolutely no scope of residual spraying in the cities.

(iv) *Personal protection* i.e. use of bednets, preferably inpregrated with pyrethroid insecticides, wearing of adequate clothes, using of insect repellants such as deet or neem seed oil can give some protection.

(v) *IEC.* Information, education and communication are important part in control procedures. Here, the term malignant malaria should first be removed. This term creates confusion in the mind of the people. The term has been deleted from the modern text books and literature. It is to be remembered that we shall have to live with malaria in foreseable future. We must not be afraid of the ancient foe. Bravely we shall have to face the situation. Fight against malaria is to be continued and every member of the society should participate.

Chapter - 9
Geographic Information System (GIS) in the Management of Urban Malaria

*Indrani Kar**

Abstract

Malaria essentially thought to be a rural problem, has been observed to be on the rise in urban areas. The urban areas with higher incidence of malaria along with unabated growth in the urban settlement has given rise to the urgent need for newer methodologies to assess the situation. Malaria has been considered to be a local phenomenon, intensity of its transmission, prevalence and distribution of parasites are determined by local malariogenic conditions, which is said to differ between different localities, even between two streets in the same locality. Moreover, the developmental activities in recent years have brought in major topographical changes in the ecosystem. Therefore, it is essential to assess the situation for the spatial distribution of malaria based on the malariogenic factors responsible for its resurgence or increase and decline in incidence. This calls for a new approach and the GIS approach for understanding the spatial pattern of the disease and gaining insight towards developing a 'spatial strategy' for urban malaria control and prevention is attractive and rewarding.

In general the GIS would be of great help in understanding the area specific malaria receptivity and vulnerability at macro and micro level and would aid in the institution of various area specific control measures at the appropriate time, saving manpower, material and money.

Introduction

Measures to improve health and the quality of life are gaining greater attention together with the need to protect and improve the environment. One of the most important questions asked in the

* Vidhyasagar College for Women, 39, Shankar Ghosh Lane, Kolkata-700006

public and environmental health today concerns the type of instrument that can be used to device quick, reliable and scientifically valid methods for rapid assesment of the situation in orders to assist in health research, planning, monitoring and evaluation of health programmes.

Malaria is recognised as one of the most prevalent and debilitating tropical diseases with more than 2.1 billion people at risk of infection (WHO, 1993).

The objectives of the WHO Global Strategy (1993) are to prevent morality and to reduce morbidity, social and economic loss due to the diseases through the progressive improvement and strengthening of local and national capabilities for malaria control. It has four basic technical elements.

(i) to provide early diagnosis and prompt treatment

(ii) to plan and implement selective and sustainable preventive measures including vector control

(iii) to detect early, contain and prevent epidemics and

(iv) to strengthen local capabilities in basic and applied research to permit and promote the regular assessment of malaria situation, in particular, the ecological, social and economic determinants of the disease.

The strategy calls for the rational use of existing and future tools to control malaria. It recognizes that malaria related problems vary enormously from epidemiological, ecological, social and operational viewpoints and that sustainable cost effective control must therefore be based on local analysis. Urban areas with high incidence of malaria along with unabated growth in the urban settlement has given rise to the urgent need for newer methodologies to assess the situation.

Malaria is considered as a local phenomenon, intensity of its transmission, prevalence and distribution of parasites are determined by the local malariogenic conditions, which differs from village to village, city to city and even between adjoining lanes/localities. More over the developmental activities in recent years have brought in major topographical changes in the erstwhile established ecosystem. Therefore, it is essential to assess the situation for spatial distribution of malaria based on the malariogenic factors responsible for its resurgence or increase and decline in the incidence. This calls for a new approach.

GIS may be defined as an automated information system based on the methodology of geographical data base management and query. The GIS approach for understanding the spatial pattern of the disease and gaining insight towards developing a 'spatial strategy' for urban malaria control and prevention and surely it will be rewarding.

Malaria in India was essentially a rural problem. Thus, during the launching of National Malaria Control Programme (NMCP) in 1953 and National Malaria Eradication Programme (NMEP) in 1958, no proper attention was given to tackle the urban malaria problem. Malaria in urban areas showed gradual increase (NMEP in depth evaluation, 1970). Moreover the rapid rate of developmental activities particularly in the periurban areas have resulted in the tropical aggregation of labour force from various parts of the country. Besides the urban pull have also resulted in the formation of new slums and also the expansion of the older.

Anopheles stephensi is the well established vector of major urban areas. The preferred breeding sites of this species have been found to be mainly intradomestic habitats of which overhead tanks, well, household receptacles and construction curing pits are most important (Kar *et al.* 1996). Under UMS (Urban Malaria Scheme) weekly chemical treatment of all the potential breeding sources is recommended in addition to biological control. Owing to the operational problems related to the treatment of sources, many are left untreated making the whole programme ineffective. The problem of insecticide resistance of vectors is also a cause of concern.

Studies on the alternative environment friendly methods for control of vectors by using larvivorous fishes, mosquito proofing of breeding sources through proper health education, community participation, intersectarial co-ordination have indicated promising results (Kar *et al.* 1997).

The understanding about malaria through GIS will be based on the quantitative and qualitative data at the macro and micro lavels on various malariogenic factors/parameters. The information base can be built on the spatially referred data on.

*** Urban area map with wards/divisions**

*** Epidemiological parameters-**

- Disease prevalence and distribution (wardwise/streetwise/ housewise)-Type/% distribution/deaths recorded etc.

- susceptibility status of different antimalarials.
- Relapsing pattern.

*** Entomological parameters-**

- Mosquito-density (adult and larval), types and distribution
- Vector density (adult and larval) seasonally recorded, adult resting habitat, larval breeding preferences etc. Biting pattern, vectorial capacity, resistance towards insecticides etc.

*** Geographical parameters-**

- Soil
- Elevation/contour map of the area
- Ground water table
- Meteorological informations - *viz.* Temperature, humidity, rainfall etc.

*** Demographic parameters-**

- Population density and distribution
- Literacy level/ percentage/distribution
- Socio-economic representation
- Housing pattern/presence of slums
- vulnerability movement of population/business activity etc.

*** Urban fascilities-**

- Road and transport network
- Drainage/sewarage net work and their conditions
- Water supply net work
- Construction activity, labour force presence, records on malaria etc.
- Industrial activity
- Health care fascilities, Govt./private, Hospitals/Nursing homes etc.
- Private doctors
- Medicine shops

*** Others-**

- Human cattle ratio
- Municipal infrastructure, men, material and budget
- Other relevent sociological factor that may have bearing on the control and / or prevention of the disease.

The information on the above can be collected as far as practicable at the macro and micro level and represented in the map [some (Fig. 1-6) representative maps from studies taken up in Dindigul municipality, Tamil Nadu, earlier is given here for better understanding]. The different types of maps thus created are overlayed one above the other for bringing out a clearcut correlation between the various parameters. This will be of real use for proper understanding regarding the disease and its causes, thereby aiding in the institution of area specific control measures in the shortest possible time. The wastage of money, manpower, energy can be regulated with their rational use. The data can be updated at regular intervals. This may be very much useful for future prediction and prevention of malaria epidemics in urban areas with encouraging results. The data generated can also be used for understanding and management of various other allied diseases saving large amount of man power, equipment and money.

Reference

- Who, (1993). Report of a WHO study group on the implementation of the Global plan of action for malaria control 1993-2000, *WHO Technical Report* series 839, Geneva, WHO.
- "Indepth evaluation committee Report" issued by the Directorate of *NMEP*, Delhi, 1970.
- Kar, Indranil, Alex Eapen and K. John Ravindran (1996). Domestic breeding sources and their contribution in *Anopheles stephensi* breeding in Dindigul, Tamil Nadu, *Indian J. Malariol*, **33(4):** 191-199.
- Kar, Indranil, Alex Eapen, K. John Ravindran, R. K. Chandrahas and V.P. Sharma (1997). Anopheline breeding in intra domestic sources and their management in Chennai, Tamil Nadu, *Indian J. Malariol*, (Accepted).

Fig. 1
Wardwise Map of Dindigul Municipality
(Classified according to average api of 1993 and 1994)

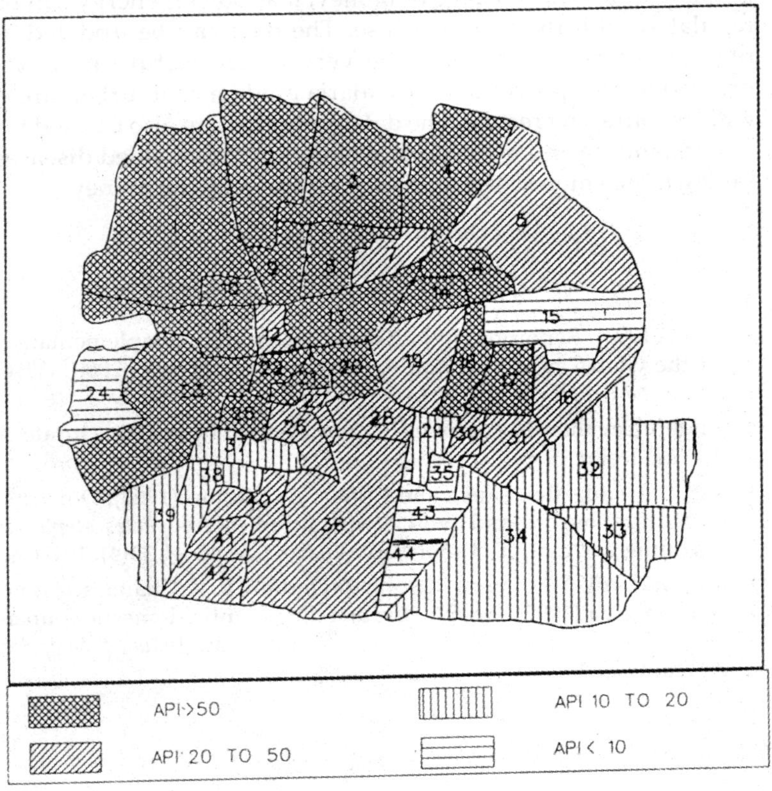

Fig. 2

Wardwise Map of Dindigul Municipality

(Classified According to Anopheline Breeding Potential)

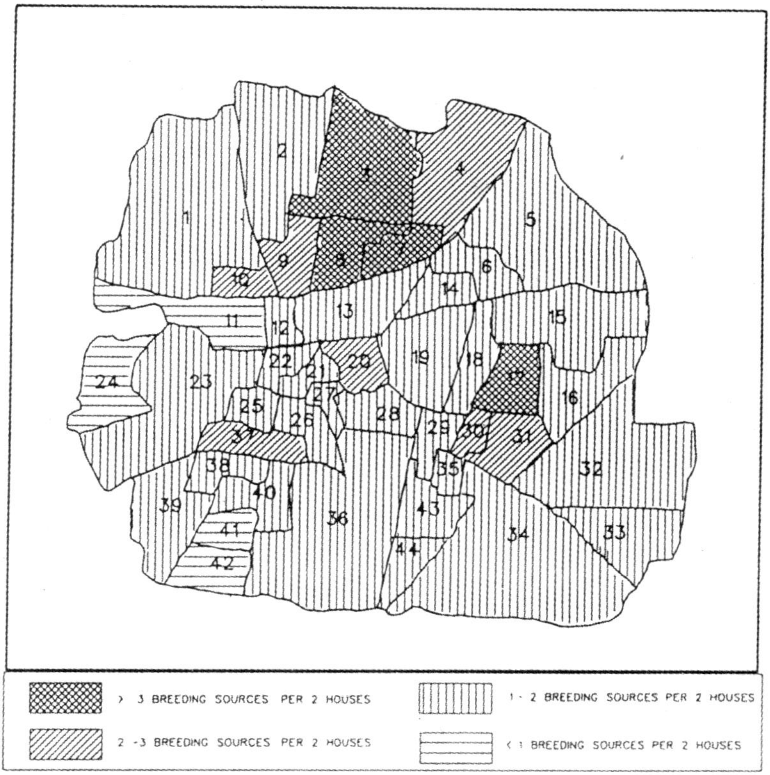

Fig. 3
Wardwise Map of Dindigul Municipality
(Classified According to Aedes Breeding Potential)

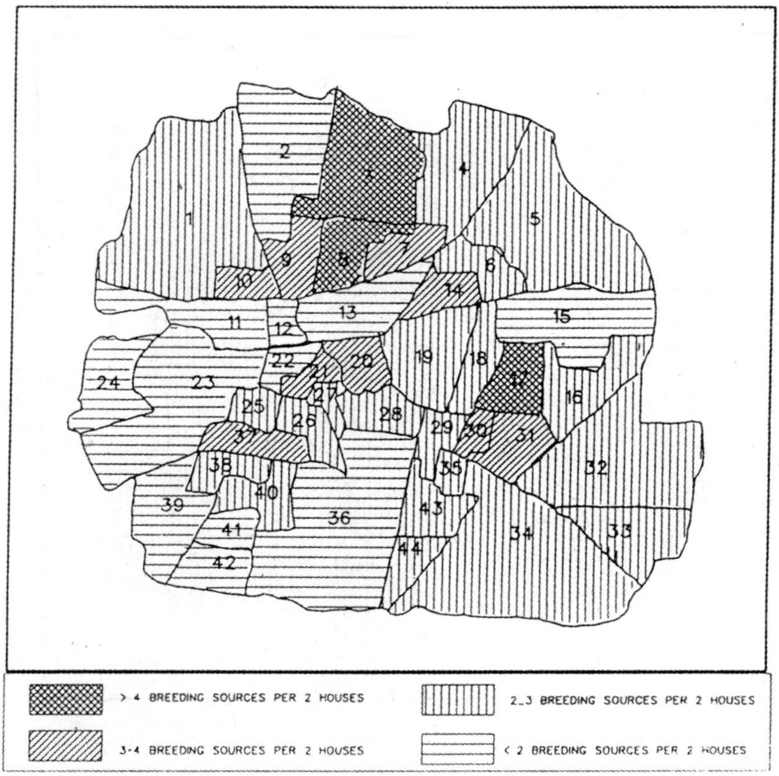

Fig. 4

Wardwise Map of Dindigul Municipality

(Classified According to Culex Bredding Potential)

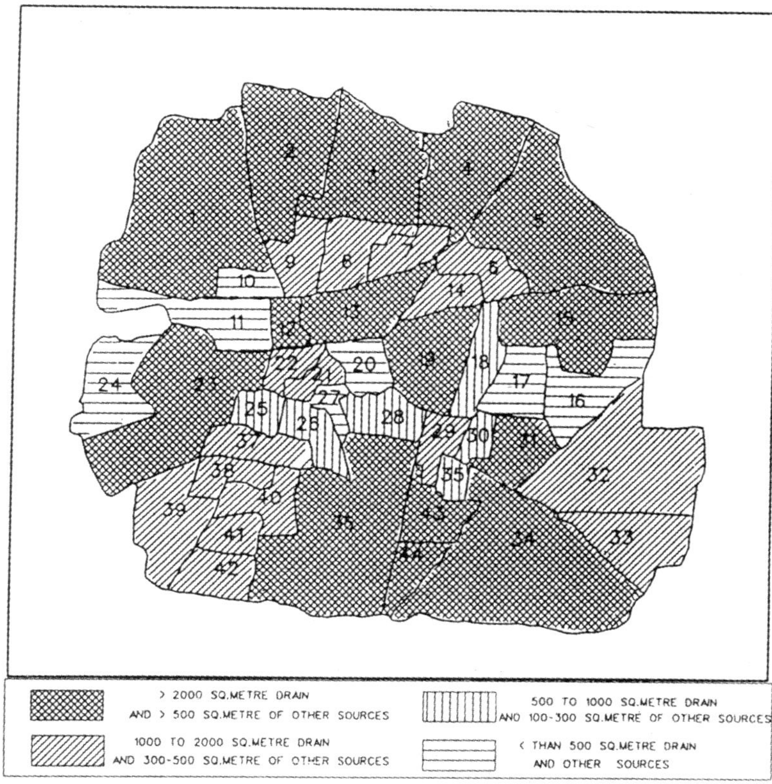

Fig. 5

Wardwise Map of Dindigul Municipality

(Classified According to Population Density)

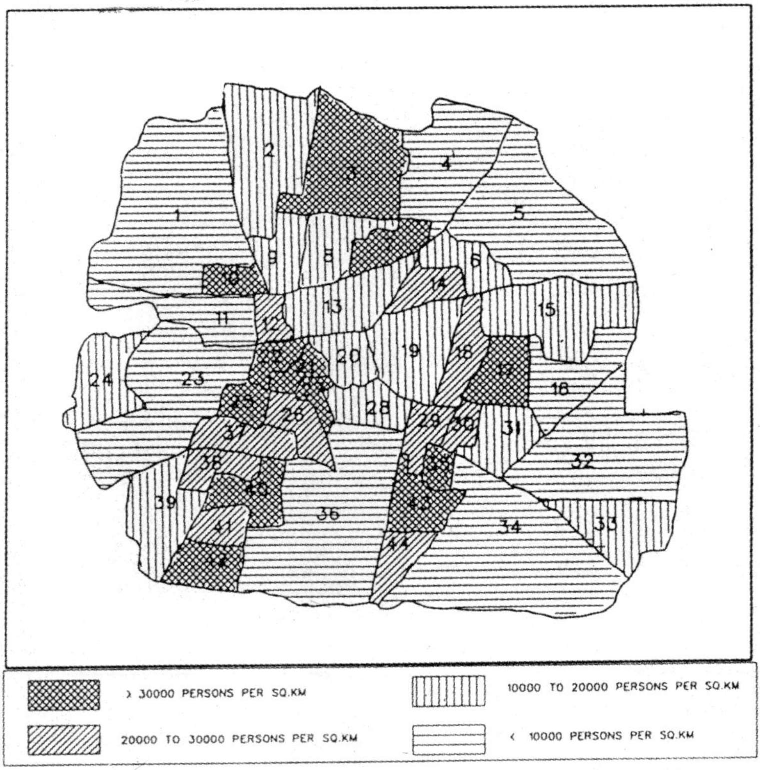

Fig. 6

Wardwise Map of Dindigul Municipality

(Classified According to Vulnerability)

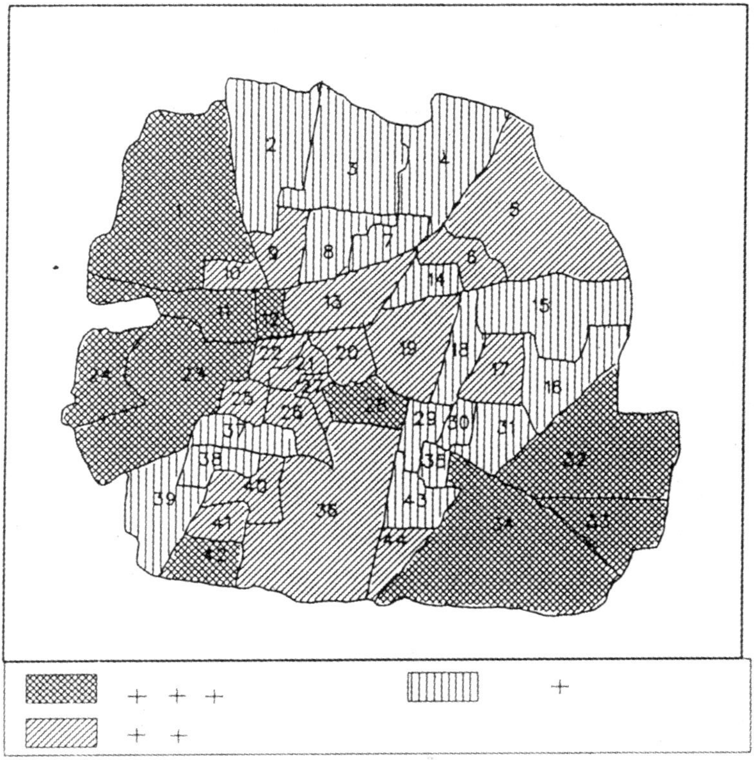

Chapter 10

Biological Vector and Sexuality in the Genus *Trypanosoma* (*Trypanozoon*)

A.K. Sarkar, K.K. Chaki** and K.K. Misra****

Abstract

There is no direct evidence that trypanosomes have sexual phases, although recent studies on iso-enzyme analyses of African trypanosomes have revealed that these populations are in Hardy-Weinberg equilibrium. In the absence of cytological evidence for sex, the accumulated data suggest that both meiosis and syngamy occur during the development of Trypanosoma (Trypanozoon) brucei in its biological vector (Glossina spp.). T. (T.) evansi is regarded as an asexual species (agamospecies) as it has no developmental phases in any kind of vector. Although being the closest relative of human sleeping sickness trypanosome, T. (T.) evansi do not exhibit any sign of sexuality probably because of its long isolation from its African relatives. Absense of sexual stages in surra trypanosome may be due to the absence of a true biological vector, the presence of which might have influenced human trypanosomes to have sexual stages. It is probable that the biological vectors provide favourable situation for possible sexual reproduction and thus contribute to the evolution of sexuality in this group.

Introduction

Syngamy or sex means fusion of two genomes, usually carried by gametes. This kind of reproduction always involves reduction usually by the process of meiosis. Evolution of sex and its consequences are a matter of deep intellectual puzzles (Stearns, 1987). Sexually reproducing species may have distinct male and female or different mating types.

* *Department of Zoology, Vivekananda College, Thakurpukur, Kolkata 700063.*

** *Department of Zoology, City College, 102/1 Raja R. M. Sarani, Kolkata 700009.*

*** *Department of Zoology, R. B. C. College, Naihati 743 165, India.*

Parasitic protozoans are a bunch of fascinating animals as different modes of reproduction are found in them. Parasitic ameobas are exclusively asexual, while the ciliates multiply both sexually and asexually. Similar practice is also found among the haemosporeans. Flagellates normally reproduce through binary fission. However, in recent times, sexuality has been suspected to be present in some species of *Trypanosoma*. Although, there is no direct evidence for sexuality in this haemoflagellate, experiments with kDNA (Ellis, 1986) and RFLPs (Turner *et al.*, 1990) strongly support the contention of covert sex in this group of parasites as proposed by Hurst *et al.* (1992).

Life cycle of many parasites is associated with insect vectors. Parasite-vector association is very much important in maintaining the different life stages, especially the sexual stages, which develop in the biological vector. Normally, a parasitic protozoon performs its asexual reproduction in the vertebrate host and sexual reproduction in the vector and is termed as heteroxenous parasite. Therefore, a biological vector plays a key role in the completion of life cycle of the parasite as well as in spreading of the disease. This association results in developing a synchronous adjustment among them and reached a perfection of parasitic adaptation. In some cases, absence of a vector in a landscape may cause extermination of the parasite in that area. The unique role of biological vector in disease transmission can be best studied in landscape epidemiology. The disease that is transmitted by a biological vector is often referred to as vector-borne disease, and it also indicates a much older association between the parasite and the vector than between the parasite and its vertebrate host.

In this article, an attempt has been made to review the scenario for the existence of sexuality in trypanosome parasite and its relationship with the biological vector. The members of the genus *Trypanosoma (Trypanozoon)* are the most pathogenic haemoflagellate of human and other mammals. Most of the species of this subgenus are transmitted by the tsetse fly (biological vector), while few are mechanically transmitted. Sexuality in these trypanosomes in relation to biological vectors is assessed.

Sexuality in protozoa

Most of the parasitic protozoons reproduce by asexual method, while some of them also exhibit sexual reproduction. Analysis of the allelic variations in seventy one isolates of *Naegleria lovaniensis* using isoenzyme markers showed that most of the loci were close to Hardy-Weinberg equilibrium suggesting segregation and free recombination between alleles (Pernin *et. al.*, 1992). However, no signs of meiosis or nuclear fusion have been observed (Vickerman, 1993). It is a known fact that different species of *Plasmodium* practise both sexual and asexual reproduction. Sexual reproduction occurs in stomach of the female anopheline mosquito, where fusion of microgametes with macrogametes results in the formation of zygote. Sexuality has also been reported in hypermastigid flagellates (e.g. *Triconympha* sp.) (Noble and Noble, 1982) as well as in ciliates (e.g. *Nyctotherus* sp.) (Smyth, 1994).

Hoare (1966, 1972) classified mammalian trypanosomes in two sections, Stercoraria (develop in hind gut of the insect vector) and Salivaria (develop in mid gut and salivary gland of insect vector). Members of the subgenus *Trypanozoon* belong to the latter group. Most of the salivarian *Trypanosoma (Trypanozoon)* are transmitted by tsetse fly (heteroxenous), while few like *T. (T.) evansi, T. (T.) equiperdum* and *T. (T.) equinum* have no biological vector (monoxenous), and are transmitted mechanically. Earlier it was thought that trypanosomes are agamospecies and exhibit no sexual stages in their life cycle. Maynard-Smith (1986) has regarded existence of completely asexual eukaryotic organism as 'evolutionary scandal'. Recently some evidence is emerging for the existence of sexual process in this group. Despite the lack of cytological evidence for sex, isoenzyme analysis of African trypanosome stock reveals that the population is in Hardy-Weinberg equilibrium suggestive of diploidy and mating (Tait, 1983).

Experiment using isoenzyme marker, RFLPs of undefined single copy genes, and RFLPs of characterized gene loci are suggestive of occurrence of recombination in African trypanosomes (*Trypanozoon*) (Turner *et al.*, 1990). Vickerman (1993) claimed that both meiosis and syngamy occur during the development of the parasite in the tsetse fly. No cytological evidence of recombination has been detected in *T. brucei*, and accordingly Tait *et al.* (1996) concluded that *T. brucei* is able to self fertilize in the presence of dissimilar stock. Komba *et al.* (1997) speculated the *T. b. rhodesiense* stocks evolve locally through frequent genetic exchange with their sympatric *T. b. brucei* stocks. All these evidence point towards existence of sexuality in trypanosomes, which is clandestine in nature (Hurst *et al.*, 1992). *T. (T.) evansi*, a closely related species of *T. b. brucei* is mechanically transmitted by the species of *Tabanus* and *Stomoxys* (Hoare, 1972). This parasite has no cyclical development and has no opportunity for mating. So this is a purely asexual species (Vickerman, 1993).

Vector and sexuality

Most of the members of subgenus *Trypanozoon* are transmitted by tsetse fly in the tsetse belt of Africa. The development of the parasite in the species of *Glossina* is completed in the anterior station with the formation of metacyclic forms. This subgenus is divided into two subgroups—*brucei* and *evansi*. *Glossina* transmits the subgroup *brucei,* while the *evansi* is transmitted mechanically or by contact. Sexual stages are suggestive in the former but absent in the latter.

Trypanosoma brucei is the only kinetoplastid known to undergo genetic exchange and it is likely that this process cannot evolve by itself (Gibson and Stevens, 1999; Gibson, 2001). However, phylogenetic tree constructed from 18s rRNA gene sequence reveals no clues to the existence of genetic exchange in trypanosomes other than salivaria (Gibson, 2001). Tibayrenc and Ayala (1999) remarked that from the evolutionary standpoint, the impact of sex appears to be greater in African than American trypanosomes. According to them, trypanosomes exhibit a basically clonal population structure, with occasional genetic exchange or hybridization and show discrete evolutionary lineages. Earlier, Tait *et al.* (1996) concluded that, as no evidence of recombination is detected, *T. brucei* may undergo self-fertilization within the vector.

Most of the authors are of opinion that high rate of antigenic variation in *T. brucei* is associated with genetic exchange, because a large proportion of the genome is devoted to variant antigen genes. It is found that biparental inheritance of kDNA in *T. brucei* takes place and genetic exchange enhances the heterogeneity of the kinetoplast DNA minicircles (Gibson, 2001). Turner (1997) observed that antigenic variation in *T. brucei* are several orders of magnitude lower in syringe-passage clones than fly-transmitted lines. It is shown that the reduction in the rate of antigenic switching in syringe-passage infection is reversible in fly-transmitted lines. Such reversible antigenic switching is unlikely to be caused by mutation, but the mechanism is still unknown.

Thus it is observed that the presence of a biological vector enhances genetic exchange in *T. brucei*. This genetic exchange may have developed either through self-fertilization or cross-fertilization. During epidemic spread of the disease the parasite population becomes clonal and this condition promotes self-fertilization leading to increase in heterozygosity within the clonal population and exhibits departure from Hardy-Weinberg equilibria and linkage disequilibria. Every time each vector-borne epidemic leads to the establishment of new endemic foci with new genetic equilibria. Clonality in *T. brucei* shows epidemic population structure. In such cases a particular clone, having specific genotype, dominates over other clones within a restricted ecological niche. In old endemic foci, multiple genotypes are present in the population and tsetse flies supposed to be infected with mixtures of stocks and both self and cross-fertilization may take place allowing the development of new generations with different allelic recombination. All these possible mechanisms may occur when a vector is present.

High level of antigenic variation in *T. brucei* allows the parasite to continue life cycle by evading antigenic challenge of the host. In such cases a disease may turn into a chronic one. Lack of antigenic variability in pathogenic parasite leads to the termination of life either of the host or of the parasite. Antigenic variability is achieved by the parasite during its course of evolution. *Trypanosoma (Trypanozoon) evansi* produces surra disease, which is very much acute in all the experimental animals (Misra *et al.*, 1976, Biswas *et al.*, 2001) as well as in natural infections and ultimately reaches a fatal end.

Being the closest relative to human sleeping sickness trypanosome, *T. (T.) evansi* do not exhibit any sign of sexuality probably of its long isolation from its African relatives and from the tsetse vector. Geographical isolation of *T. (T.) evansi* from the tsetse belt might have some effect on the sexuality and antigenic variation in this haemoflagellate. It is to be mentioned that very low percent of short-stumpy trypomastigote form of *T. (T.) evansi* is occasionally found in the blood. And only this form of trypanosome is capable of developing in the vector. Mathur (1971) provided experimental demonstration that pleomorphic variants of *T. (T.) evansi* can have a cycle of development in *Glossina morsitans.* This evidence points to the existence of potentiality of *T. (T.) evansi* to perform cyclical transmission and probability of developing sexuality. Among the salivarian species of the subgenus *Trypanozoon,* only the members of the *brucei*-subgroup have circumstantial evidence of sexuality, but not in the members of the *evansi*-subgroup, and the difference between them is the involvement of the biological vector in the former but not in the latter.

Discussion

The foregoing evidence clearly indicates that cyclical development of kinetoplastid haemoflagellates in the vector provides an opportunity for mating. The only trypanosomatid so far proved to undergo genetic exchange is *T. brucei* (Gibson and

Stevens, 1999; Gibson, 2001). Analogous mating experiments have been attempted with other *Trypanosoma* species but without any success. The pleomorphic stumpy form of *T. brucei* is preadapted for the midgut of *Glossina* and, therefore, has an opportunity for further development in the vector host. Likewise, the metacyclic form of this species, found in the salivary gland of the tsetse fly, is preadapted for vertebrate host and can invade it easily. In both cases, the preadaptive features include physiological and antigenic characteristics. Thus the possible site of meiosis and syngamy of *T. brucei* is the salivary gland of *Glossina* (Vickerman, 1993). Antigenic variation is one of the characteristic that shared by the salivarian *Trypanozoon*. The large proportion of the genome engaged in producing various antigens provides a possible role for genetic exchange, which may enhance the potential diversity (Gibson, 2001). Although *T. evansi* exhibits antigenic variations, no sexual stages or evidence of sexuality has so far been observed or obtained. Thus it is surprising that without any genetic exchange, how so much of antigenic variations are maintained by this species. The occurrence of stumpy form of *T. evansi* is very rare. This might be one of the plausible reasons for the failure of *T. evansi* to be established within a biological vector, and as such no chance for mating.

Although, on the basis of their DNA content, it was formerly thought that metacyclic stages of *T. (T.) b. brucei* were haploid, it is now thought that trypanosomes are diploid throughout their life cycle, but may contain variable amount of DNA (Ash, 1990). Occurrence of variable amount of DNA in different stages of life cycle can be explained by the presence of sexual process, which involve meiosis and syngamy. However, the orders of these processes have not yet been worked out.The experiment with kDNA proves the presence of recombination, which is only possible in meiotic cell division. Again, determination of ploidy in trypanosomes shows that they may be of haploid, diploid or polyploid. Therefore, it is obvious that some fusion systems are present in the life cycle as well as reduction division system in these haemoflagellates.

Thus it can be summarized that some members of the subgenus *Trypanozoon* of the genus *Trypanosoma* (viz., *brucei*-subgroup) show the existence of genetic exchange, which takes place during their development within the vector. The members of the entire *evansi*-subgroup, on the other hand, fail to exhibit sexuality as the parasite does not enjoy invertebrate biological vector.

References

- Ash, C. (1990). Editorial. *Parasitol. Today,* **6**: 61.
- Biswas. D., Choudhury, A. and Misra, K. K. (2001). Histopathology of *Trypanosoma (Trypanozoon) evansi* infection in Bandicoot rat. I. Visceral organs. *Exptl. Parasitol.,* **99**: 148-159.
- Ellis, D. S. (1986). Sex and the single trypanosome. *Parasitol. Today,* **2**: 184-185.
- Gibson, W. (2001). Sex and evolution in trypanosomes. *Int. J. Parasitol.,* **31**: 643-647.
- Gibson, W. and Stevens, J. (1999). Genetic exchange in the trypanosomatidae. *Adv. Parasitol.,* **43**: 1-46.
- Hoare, C. A. (1996). The classification of mammalian trypanosomes. Ergebn. *Mikrobiol,* **39**: 43-57.
- Hoare, C. A. (1972). *The Trypanosomes of Mammals.* A Zoological Monograph. Blackwell, Oxford.
- Hurst, L. D., Hamilton, W. D. and Ladle, R. (1992). Covert sex. *Trends Ecol. Evol.,* **7**: 144-145.
- Komba, E. K., Kibona, S. N., Ambwene, A. K., Stevens, J. R. and Gibson, W. C. (1997). Genetic diversity among *Trypanosoma brucei rhodesiense* isolates from Tanzania. *Parasitology,* **115**: 571-579.
- Mathur, S. C. (1971). Cultivation of a pleomorphic variant of *Trypanosoma (Trypanozoon) evansi* and its transmission by *Glossina morsitans. Trans. R. Soc. trop. Med. Hyg.,* **65**: 427.
- Maynard-Smith, J. (1986). Contemplating life without sex. *Nature, Lond.,* **324**: 300-301.
- Misra, K. K. Ghose, M. and Choudhury, A. (1976). Experimental transmission of *T. evansi* to chicken. *Acta Protozool.,* **15**: 381-386.
- Noble, E. R. and Noble, G. A. (1982). Parasitology. *The Biology of Animal Parasites.* 5th ed., Lea and Febiger, Philadelphia.
- Pernin, P., Ataya, A. and Cariou, M. L. (1992). Genetic structure of natural populations of the free-living amoeba *Naegleria lovaniensis.* Evidence for sexual reproduction. *Heredity,* **68**: 173-181.
- Smyth, J. D. (1994). *Animal Parasitology.* 3rd ed. Cambridge University Press, Cambridge.
- Stearns, S. C. (ed.) (1987). *The evolution of sex and its consequences.* Birkhauser-Verlag, Basel.
- Tait, A. (1983). Sexual processes within the Kinetoplastida. *Parasitology,* **86**: 29-57.
- Tait, A., Buchanan, N., Hide, G. and Turner, C. M. R. (1996). Self-fertilization in *Trypanosoma brucei. Mol. Biochem. Parasitol.,* **76**: 31-42.
- Tibayrenc, M. and Ayala, F. J. (1999). Evolutionary genetics of *Trypanosoma* and *Leishmania. Microbes infect.,* **1**: 465-472.
- Turner, C. M. R. (1997). The rate of antigenic variation in fly-transmitted and syringe-passaged infections of *Trypanosoma brucei. FEMS Microbiology lett.,* **153**: 227-231.

- Turner, C. M. R., Sternberg, J., Buchanan, N., Smith, E., Hide, G. and Tait, A. (1990). Evidence that the mechanism of gene exchange in *Trypanosoma brucei* involves meiosis and syngamy. *Parasitology,* **101**: 377-386.
- Vickerman, K. (1993). Natural selection and the life cycles of protozoan parasites. *Proc. zool. Soc., Calcutta, Haldane Comm. Vol.,* **41-52**.

Chapter - 11
House Dust Mite Allergy: An Environmental Enigma

** Goutam Kumar Saha*

Abstract

House dust allergy is a fairly common problem among sensitive individuals, resulting in various types of allergic manifestations like allergic rhinitis, atopic eczema, bronchial asthma etc. About 4% of the world population reportedly suffer from different types of allergic disorders. In India, 10 million people suffer from asthma and another 15 million from other recurrent allergic diseases. The nasobronchial passage of susceptible individuals is sensitive to various external substances namely pollens, moulds, feathers, furs, animal danders, dust etc. repeated exposure to which may trigger off allergic manifestations.

Introduction

House dust is a complex mixture of substances of plant and animal origin and consists of animal and human dander, debris from wool, feathers, hairs, insects, cotton, silk, jute and synthetic fibers, carpets, beddings, furniture and upholstery. Besides, fungal spores, bacteria, microorganisms and shedding from other house hold articles also contribute to its composition. Although house dust has long been known to cause sneezing and wheezing in sensitive subjects, the exact nature of the principal allergen in house dust was unknown for quite a long time. Kern (1921) and Cooke (1922) highlighted the role of house dust in causing respiratory allergy and suggested the presence of distinct allergen in it. It was Voorhorst *et al.* (1964) who first pointed out that house dust mites belonging to the genus *Dermatophagoides* of the Family Pyroglyphidae are most potent allergen in house dust responsible for various allergic manifestations. Subsequently allergy skin tests

* Dept. of Zoology, University of Calcutta, Kolkata-700 019.

and nasal and bronchial challenge tests have clearly established that Pyroglyphid mites are chiefly responsible for house dust allergy (Voorhorst *et al.* 1964, Pepys *et al.* 1968). These findings were further confirmed by the estimation of total serum IgE level and detection of mite specific IgE antibodies present in patients sera (Aas and Johansson 1971; Dockhorn 1982; Saha *et al.* 1989 and Saha 1993). In India, Shivpuri and Agarwal (1971) first of all claimed that the mite is perhaps the sole potent allergen responsible for precipitation of attack of bronchial asthma. Since then the studies on house dust mite fauna and their probable role on the aetiopathogenesis of different allergic disorders have been reported from different parts of India (Lal *et al.* 1973; Nayar *et al.* 1974; Dar and Gupta 1979; Shivpuri 1981; Jamil and Maurya 1981; Tandon *et al.* 1988, 1990; Roy *et al.* 1987; Modak *et al.* 1991, 1995; Saha 1993, 1994, 1997 and Saha *et al.* 1989, 1995). From Calcutta, Saha (1993, 1994, 1997) and Saha *et al.* (1995) reported that more than 88% of the asthmatic patients are sensitive to *Dermatophagoides* mites as evidenced from analysis of house dust, allergy skin test and detection of allergen specific IgE antibodies by RAST method. Besides *Euroglyphus maynei, Tyrophagus putrescentiae, Acarus siro* and *Glycyphagus domesticus* are also known to produce allergens in house dust though with relatively low potency (Voorhorst and Spieksma 1973).

Mites (Arthropoda: Arachnida: Acari) are minute (0.5 to 2mm in length) and are characterised by the absence of antennae and mandibles and the presence of simple eyes, four pairs of walking legs and two pairs of specialized mouthparts- chelicerae and pedipalpi. The majority of mites are free living, but thousands of species parasitize plants and animals, infesting internal organs such as inner and middle ear, respiratory passage, skin and intestine of vertebrate species, while others serve as both reservoirs and vectors of serious pathogens (Rickettsial pox and scrub typhus). These tiny and delicate organisms exhibit extreme diversity in structure, habitat and behaviour. Among them there is a taxonomically and ecologically defined assemblage called "House Dust Mite" chiefly consisting of *Dermatophagoides* spp. They are free living and occupy every niche of the house, being more abundant in beds than elsewhere, because beds are rich in human scales on which they feed (Speaksma, 1967 and Bronswijk, 1972) and provide the ideal microclimate such as temperature and humidity etc. Among several species of *Dermatophagoides* mites, *D. pteronyssinus* and *D. farinae* are most common and ubiquitous in distribution (Wharton, 1976).

During the last few decades the mite fauna of house dust in different parts of the world has received considerable attention due to its tremendous medical importance. Review of literature revealed that extensive research work on house dust mites specially *Dermatophagoides* spp. in relation to nasobronchial allergic disorders dates back to the early 20th century. The view that mites could be held responsible for asthma was first put forward by the Italian physician Anocona Giacomo in the year 1923, on the basis of his observation on grain workers suffering from asthma and dermatitis on the neck, breast and arms. In the past, several cases of allergic diseases had been described in people handling materials heavily infested with mites. Inhalation of this allergen along with dust particles is the root cause for different allergic manifestations such as allergic rhinitis, bronchial asthma etc. In some cases the entire body of the mites, dead or alive may be the source of allergen while in others the peritrophic membrane or the faecal pellets act as the sites for the origin of allergens. It is now well documented that the allergenicity of the dust sample depends on the number/load of mites specially the Pyroglyphids contained in the dust (Saha 1994).

Mites in house dust

The mite fauna of house dust is poorly known and more than 130 species of mites have so far been isolated from the house dust samples all over the world (Zheltikova *et al.* 1985). The first report of occurrence of mites in Indian house dust came from the study of Krishna Rao *et al.* (1973) who reported a large number of Pyroglyphids in house dust. Subsequently studies on the house dust mite fauna have been conducted in different parts of the country from time to time and presence of a varying number of species of dust mites have been reported (Dixit and Mehta 1973; Gupta and Dutta Ray 1975; Dar and Gupta 1979; Rao *et al.* 1981; Maurya and Jamil 1981; Tripathi and Parikh 1983, Channa Basavanna *et al.* 1984; Tandon *et al.* 1988, Kumar *et al.* 1988 and Kumud *et al.* 1988). Dar and Gupta (1979) collected dust samples from houses of bronchial asthma patients from 19 states of India and identified mite fauna belonging to 18 families. From Karnataka, Krishna Rao *et al.* (1981) described 23 species of mites belonging to six families. Maurya *et al.* (1983) obtained 16 species and some unidentified forms from six states of India while Tripathi and Parikh (1983) reported seven species from patients' houses residing in Mumbai. Twenty species of mites under six families and two orders have been reported by Channa Basavanna *et al.* (1984) from

Bangalore. So far, to the best of our knowledge a maximum of 27 mite species distributed over 21 genera and 10 families have been reported from Punjab and Himachal Pradesh (Kumar *et al.* 1988). Kumud *et al.* (1988) reported the presence of 17 species under 14 genera and 10 families from 200 dust samples collected from Haryana. From West Bengal Tandon *et al.* (1988) identified 22 species of mites under 19 genera and 13 families from dust samples of houses of asthmatic patients of Calcutta. Modak *et al.* (1989) in a comparative study reported the presence of 54 species from three different districts of West Bengal namely 24 Parganas, Burdwan and Calcutta. Among them maximum variety were isolated from the Calcutta metropolis. Both the species of *Dermatophagoides* mites i.e. *D. farinae* and *D. pteronyssinus* are present in the house dust samples collected from different parts of India of which in most cases the later predominates (Dixit and Mehta 1973; Rao *et al.* 1981; Maurya *et al.* 1983; Tandon *et al.* 1988; Modak *et al.* 1991 and Kumud *et al.* 1988). In contrast Dar *et al.* (1973) and Jamil and Maurya (1981) reported the predominance of *D. farinae* in the dust samples collected from different states of India. However, Tripathi and Parikh (1983) noted preponderance of *D. farinae* in floor dust while *D. pteronyssinus* was predominant in bed dust.

During last 14 years, we have studied the house dust mite fauna of West Bengal. A total of 14 districts of West Bengal including Calcutta metropolis have been searched for mite fauna. The rate of occurrence was almost 90%. A total of 68 species of mites belonging to 25 families under 44 genera and 3 orders namely, Astigmata, Prostigmata and Mesostigmata have been reported including a good number of unidentified Cryptostigmatids. Among them six species appeared to be new to science while another 20 species were reported for the first time from Indian house dust samples. It is interesting to note that maximum number (47) of mite species were isolated form dust samples of Calcutta followed by 40 from Burdwan and 33 from 24 Parganas (North and South) and least (6) from Birbhum district. *D. pteronyssinus* was the most dominating mite species (Fig. 1) comprising 69% of the total mite fauna followed by *D. fairnae* (14%), *Hirstia domicola* (13%), *Malayoglyphus intermedins* (0.86%) and *Euroglyphus maynei* (0.12%). It was also observed that the bed dust samples contained higher mite densities than the corresponding bedroom floor dust samples. The incidence of 13,750 mites per gram of dust was observed from a bed dust sample collected from the Calcutta metropolis.

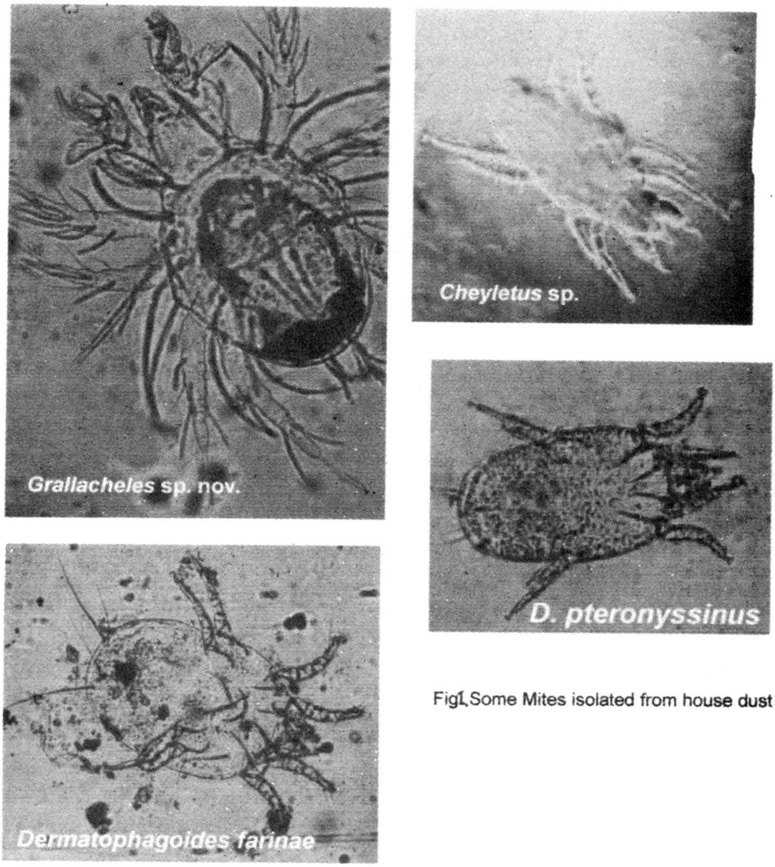

Fig1.Some Mites isolated from house dust

Seasonal abundance of mites

The population density of *Dermatophagoides* mites tends to fluctuate seasonally (Arlian *et al.* 1982). In India, the seasonal abundance of dust mite fauna is yet to be studied in a comprehensive manner. However, notable contribution in this area came from Dar *et al.* (1973) and Dar and Gupta (1979). According to them, the mite density reached the maximum in the month of August - September while it was minimum in March to May. According to Kumar *et al.* (1988) the mites were most abundant in warm season (July to October) and their density declined during hot (March to June) and cold (November to February) periods. In our study from West bengal, we found that the density of all types of mites in bed and bedroom floor dust were maximum in autumn (September to November) and lowest in monsoon (June to August).

Similar trend was also found in case of Pyroglyphids but only in bed dust sample. However, in bedroom floor dust sample density of Pyroglyphids was observed to be maximum in summer (March to May) and minimum in monsoon (June to August). It has been recognized that temperature and humidity are the two important key factors controlling mite abundance. Bronswijk (1973) and Arlian and Veselica (1981) reported that the annual periodicity is positively correlated with humidity cycle in the house. According to Spieksma *et al.* (1971) the mites are very sensitive to variations in humidity and under RH conditions lower than 70% the population stops growing. It may be concluded that a temperature of 25^{0}C-30^{0}C and RH between 65%-75% are optimum for the successful growth and multiplication of mites and any variation in these factors is detrimental and ultimately fatal to these small arthropods.

Biology and behaviour

The life cycle of *D. pteronnysinus* shows seven distinct developmental stages namely egg, larva, protonymph, resting protonymph, tritonymph, resting tritonymph and adult (Ho and Nadchtram 1984, Mutsumoto *et al.* 1986 and Modak *et al.* 2000). However, Bronswijk and Sinha (1971) earlier reported the presence of only five life stages and excluded the possibility of any resting or pharate proto and tritonymphal stages. It usually takes 14-16 days to complete the lifecycle at a temperature ranging from 25^{0}C to 33^{0}C and RH varying from 57-89%, without any deutonymphal stage (Modak *et al.* 2000). Earlier workers (Bronswijk and Sinha 1971, Ho and Nadchatram 1984) reported a longer (average 33 days) in both *D. farinae* and *D. pteronyssinus* while according to Matsumoto *et al.* (1986) the life cycle of *D. pteronyssinus* was completed in 37 days. The life cycle was faster at higher temperature but egg production is relatively less at low temperature (Furumizo 1975). On an average the egg laying capacity of females ranged from 0.6 to 1.7 per day. The life span of adult male varies from 4 - 5 weeks and the female mites lived longer than their male counterparts. On an average a female lived for 36 days, deposited 50 eggs, and copulated 4 times. Males lived for 23 days on an average, fertilizing as many as 5 females during this period. The morality rate was highest in larval stages (44%) and gradually decreased as the development progressed. Otani *et al.* (1984) reported that the density of mite population was significantly higher in old and damp houses and they were much more abundant in mattress dust than anywhere else in the house (Wharton 1976). According to Blythe (1976) light, temperature,

RH, mechanical disturbances, predation and parasitism, inter and intraspecific competition along with sufficient and right type of food are the main requirements for the successful growth and multiplication of these mites. More specifically, among different types of mattresses used, the foam mattress harbour significantly higher mite densities than conventionally used cotton mattress. This is probably due to the seldom cleaning of the former and availability of ideal micro-climatic conditions (Ho and Nadchatram 1984).

Mechanism of allergic reactions

In case of atopic patients, there is a special type of antibody called immunoglobulin E (lgE). It is a distinct class of serum protein (glycoprotein) and consists of 4 polypeptide chains. It has a typical Y shaped structure and one pair of polypeptide chain contains approximately twice as many amino acids as other pair. They are thus called as heavy and light chains respectively, the chains are held together by non-covalent forces and by covalent disulphide bridges (Fig. 2). Each polypeptide chain is marked by two distinct zones; one is called variable zone (V) or the antigen binding site and other is constant zone (C) by which they are attached to mast cells. lgE is synthesized by special kinds of cells called 'B' lymphocytes of immune system and are found attached to the surface of the mast cells and in the blood fixed to basophils or free in serum. Serum lgE levels are deemed to develop an important risk factor in allergic diseases resulting from immediate hypersensitivity. In case of healthy people the concentration of lgE is generally very low (0.004% of the total immunoglobulin) and the level gets elevated in patients with allergic disorders, suggesting thereby that quantification of serum lgE level is an important marker for the diagnosis of allergic diseases (Johansson *et al.* 1972). The discovery of this new immunoglobulin and subsequent development of new techniques to measure total lgE protein and detection of allergen specific lgE antibodies by Radio Allergo Sorbent Test (RAST) method opened a new vista for the diagnosis and treatment of various allergic diseases. In human being mast cells are found specially in lungs, the upper respiratory tract, skins, intestine etc. The cytoplasm of the mast cell is rich with some biochemical mediators like histamine, bradykinin, prostaglandin, Slow Reacting Substance of Anaphylaxis (SRS-A) etc.

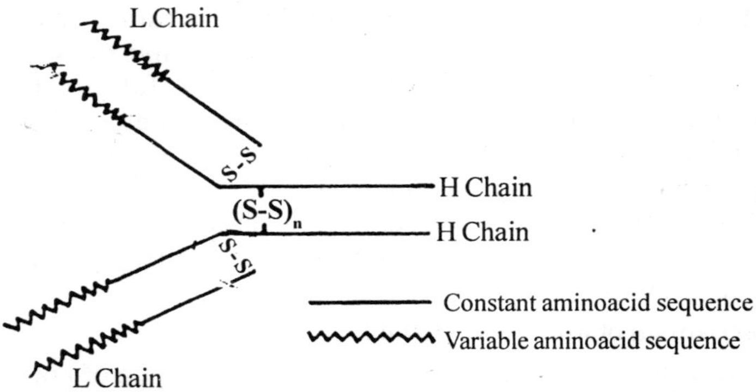

Fig. 2. Structure of an Immunoglobulin E Molecule

On initial exposure, allergens must be abundant to activate the mast cell bound lgE molecules. When the harmful allergen approaches this sensitized mast cell, the allergenic determinants get attached to the specific "V" sites of the lgE molecules on the mast cell. As a result a bridging reaction takes place which leads to the degranulation of mast cell with the release of mediators like histamine, which are actually responsible for different allergic symptoms (Fig. 3). The reaction between reagin and allergens are immunologically specific and the symptoms may appear within a couple of minutes.

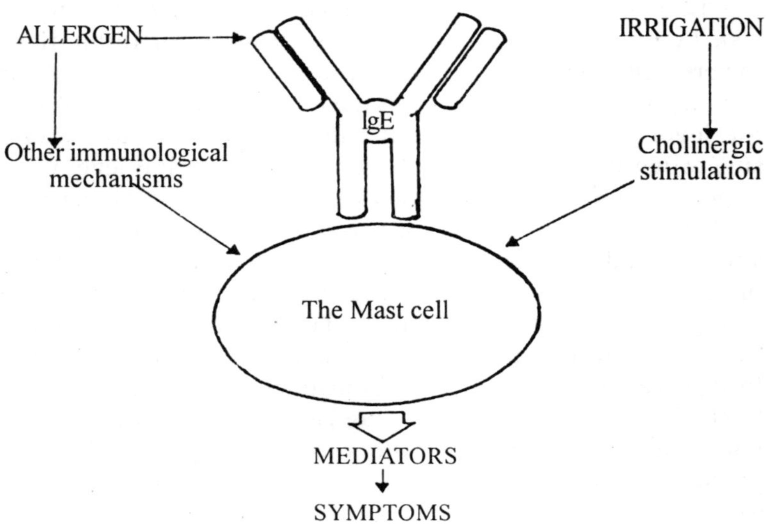

Fig. 3. Diagram Showing Mechanism of Allergic Reactions

The resulting mediators causes dialation of blood vessels and capillary permeability increases resulting in swelling. In addition they also contract the bronchial smooth muscles, swells the membrane, produces thick mucus and ultimately results in breathing troubles particularly during expiration. Externally it produces wheal and flare reactions, i.e. elevated patches with itching and surrounding redness. A similar observation is made in urticaria. Finally, histamine gives the typical symptoms of hay fever in the nose and eyes mainly sneezing, blocked nose, swollen and itching eyes.

Heredity and allergy

It has been proved that the entire immune system and the production of antibodies are governed by some genetic factors and heredity plays an important role in the development of allergic manifestations. Kjellman (1977) proved that a child with atopic parents is six times more susceptible to allergies than the children with no parental history of atopic disorders. Atopy is very high when both the parents have suffered from same diseases, affecting same organ such as skin or respiratory tract etc. The following table shows the chance of occurrence of atopy in children from parents with different degrees of atopy.

Atopy in parents	Frequency of atopy in children
1. No atopy	12.5%
2. One parent atopic	19.8%
3. Both parents atopic	42.9%
4. Both atopic with same manifestation	72.2%

Diagnosis

Effective management of allergic diseases require reliable identification of offending allergen and avoidance of that particular allergen by the patient. For this reason a detailed case history of the patient including the history of atopy is of prime importance as the case history holds a central position in allergological investigations. Sometimes, but certainly not always, it is unambiguous. In certain cases the case history can be difficult to interpret or directly misleading. Clinical diagnosis involves skin-testing, analysis of serum for total IgE and allergen specific IgE antibodies and different types of challenge tests. The diagnosis must be accurate. Doubtful test results should not be accepted. At the same time the diagnostic techniques should not put the patient at risk.

Skin testing detects reagins fixed to the mast cells in the skin and offers an important tool for allergy diagnosis. It can be performed either as a prick or scratch test or as an intracutaneous test. Among them, prick testing should at present be the form of skin testing to be recommended both for children and adults. It is highly specific from an immunological point of view and involves minimal risk. It is easy to perform and to standardize and gives little pain to the patient. The results are taken twenty minutes after testing and graded as 1^+, 2^+, 3^+, 4^+, or negative on the basis of intensity of reaction and erythema formation as compared to positive (histamine) and negative (normal saline) control as suggested by Grater *et al.* (1982). Although, intracutaneous testing is appoxiamately 10-100 times more sensitive than prick testing, more often it gives non-specific reactions and involves risk of anaphylactic shocks and also painful for the patients.

The healthy, non-atopic individual has a very low level of lgE in serum, while in many patients with atopic manifestations significantly increased lgE level are found. Thus quantification of total lgE in serum will provide information on the atopic status of the patients, confirmation of suspected atopic disease and also prediction of atopic allergy in children. To measure low level of lgE in serum sensitive RIA (Radio Immuno Assay) method have been developed such as Double Antibody technique, RIST (Radio Immuno Sorbent Test) and PRIST (Paper Radio Immuno Sorbent Test). Similarly, detection of allergen specific lgE antibodies in serum can be done by RAST (Radio Allergo Sorbent Test). The method is semi - quantitative and results are graded in a scale from 0-4. In Calcutta population, Saha *et al.* (1989) and Saha (1993) reported that 92% asthma patients showed elevated serum lgE level (above 300 IU/ml) and the mean value was significantly higher in comparison to control subjects sera ($p<<0.001$) as shown in Table 1 and Fig. 4. RAST results also indicate a higher sensitivity (85%) to house dust and house dust mites (*Dermatophagoides* spp.) either alone or in combination with each other. Among positive patients 72% showed the presence of allergen specific lgE antibodies against *D. pteronyssinus* and 89% against *D. farinae* mite antigen (Saha, 1993).

Table 1 . Serum lgE Level in Asthmatic Patients and Control Subjects

Study group	Range of lgE level	Mean lgE	Remark
Patient	55-2791 IU/ml	1002 ± 614 IU/ ml	
Control	15-120 IU/ml	56 ± 34 IU/ ml	$p<<0.001$

ANOVA (One way classified data)

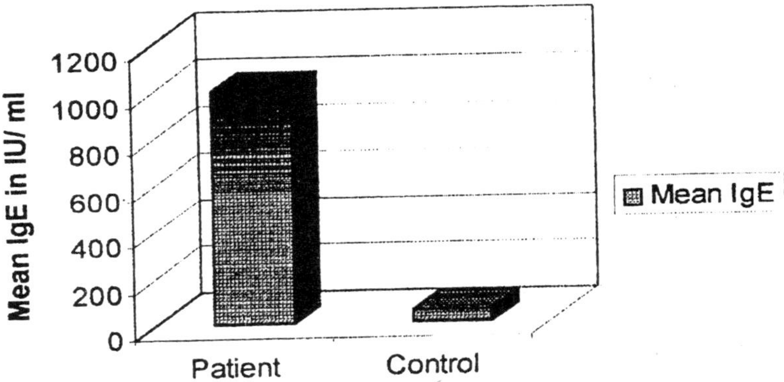

Fig. 4. Circulating IgE Levels in Asthmatic Patients Compared with their Controls

Exact allergy diagnosis is often a combination of case history and the different test methods. Thus if a patient with a positive case history of atopy presents a positive skin test as well as circulating IgE antibodies for a specific allergen this will give a strong indication of a clinically important allergy to that particular allergen.

Control measures

There is no simple and effective way to cure mite borne allergic diseases, but the symptoms may be relieved or minimized and in best cases eliminated with the adoption of combination of suitable preventive as well as curative measures. If the patient can be maintained relatively free of symptoms, the chances of increasing the tolerance with time improve and the risk of developing new allergies minimizes. However, the tendency towards spontaneous development of tolerance varies markedly with age and with the type of symptoms and allergens.

Preventive measures

1. Proper sanitation, hygiene and a general cleanliness of the bed and bedroom should be recommended.
2. Avoidance of suspected offending allergens as far as practicable.
3. House dust mites seem to thrive best on human skin scales: supply of food materials to the mites should be restricted.
4. Periodic shaking of bedroll and frequent washing of bed sheets and blankets should be done.
5. Avoid use of carpets, foam mattresses and other padded furniture in the patient's bedroom.

6. Reduction of dampness and non-availability of moisture drastically reduces mite population.
7. To reduce mite population, various acaricides have been recommended such as benzyl benzoate, pirimiphos methyl or lindane. Lindane impregnated in cloth @ 10 gm/ m^2 can effectively kill cent percent mites when exposed to it for 155 days.

Curative measures

For curative treatment of asthma the use of some bronchodialator such as salbutamol, sodium cromoglycate etc. in the form of spray, tablet or injection are recommended. The sprays are of common use to give immediate relief. In case of severe asthma steroids may be used while for urticarial rash, the use of antihistaminic or other anti-allergic drugs give the best result. Since house dust mite allergens cause asthma in sensitized individuals desensitization with mite extracts has also been recommended.

The harm caused by house dust mites are enormous which affects the socio - economic condition of the individual. Allergy is a disabling disease, some times dangerous or even fatal. It is therefore recommended that proper identification of the causative allergen and subsequently the reduction of load of this offending allergens from the patients environment may be helpful for the prophylactic management of various allergic disorders.

References

- Aas, K. and Johansson, S. G. O. (1971). The radioallergosorbent test in the in-vitro diagnosis of multiple reaginic allergy. *J. Allergy Clin Immunol.* 48 : 134-142.
- Ancona, G.(1923). Asma epidemico da pediculoides ventricosus. *Policlinico,* 30 : 45-70.
- Arlian, L. G., Bernstein, I. L. and Gallagher, J. S. (1982). The prevalence of house dust mites, *Dermatophagoides* sp. and associated environmental conditions in homes in Ohio, *J. Allergy Clin. Immunol.* 69: 527-532.
- Arlian, L. G. and Veselica, M. M. (1981). Re-evaluation of the humidity requirments of the house dust mite *Dermatophagoides farinae. J. Med. Entomol.* 18(4) : 351-356.
- Blythe, M. E. (1976). Some aspects of the ecological study of the house dust mites. *Brit. J. Dis. Chest.* 70 : 3-31.

- Bronswijk, J. E. M. H. Van. and Sinha, R. N. (1971). Pyroglyphid mites (Acari) and house dust allergy. *J. Allergy* 47: 31-52.
- Bronswijk, J. E. M. H. Van. (1972). Food preference of Pyroglyphid house dust mites. *Neth. J. Zool.* 22(3): 335-340.
- Bronswijk, J. E. M. H. Van. (1973). *Dermatophagoides pteronyssinus* (Trouessart, 1897) in mattress and floor dust in a temperate climate (Acari : Pyroglyphidae). *J. Med. Entomol.* 10 : 63-70.
- Channa Basavanna, G. P., Krishna Rao, N. S. and Ranganath, H. R. (1984). An improved method of isolation and counts of mites in a house dust sample. *Ind. J. Acar.* 9 : 89-94.
- Cooke, R. A. (1922). Studies in specific hypersensitiveness, IV. New etologic factors in bronchial asthma. *J. Immunol,* 7 : 147-162.
- Dar, N., Menon, M. P. S., Shivpuri, D. N. and Gupta, V. K. (1973). The mite fauna of Indian house dust. *Aspects of Allergy and Applied Immunology* 6 : 51-60.
- Dar, N. and Gupta, V. K. (1979). Studies on house dust mites of India and their role in causation of bronchial asthma and allergic rhinitis; Part I : *The mites. Oriental Insects* 13 : 261-298.
- Dixit, I. P. and Mehta, R. S. (1973). Prevalence of *Dermatophagoides* species in India and its role in the causation of bronchial asthma. *J. Assoc. Physicians India* 21 : 31-37.
- Dockhorn, R. (1982) Using the RAST with an overview of clinical significance. *Ann. Allergy* 49 : 1-8.
- Furumizo, R. T. (1975). Laboratory observations on the life history and biology of the American house dust mite *Dermatophagoides farinae* (Acarina : Pyroglyphidae). *Calif. Vector News* 22 : 49-60.
- Grater, W. C. , Dockhorn, R., Boggs, P. and Don, R. L. (1982). Report of the American College of Allergists' Committee on standardization of allergic extract. *Ann. Allergy* 49 : 49-54.
- Gupta, S. K. and Datta Roy, R. K. (1975). Occurrence of house dust mites in West Bengal (India). *Newls. Zool. Surv. India* 1(3) : 48-50.
- Ho, T. M. and Nadchatram, M. (1984). Life cycle and longevity of *Dermatophagoides pteronyssinus,* Trouessart (Acarina : Astigmata : Pyroglyphidae) in a tropical laboratory. *Tropical Biomedicine* 1 : 159-162.
- Jamil, Z. and Maurya, K. R. (1981). Explotion of the requisites for the mass culture of *Dermatophagoides farinae.* In : *Contributions in Acarology in India* (Channa Basavanna, G. P. ed.) 27 : 111-115.
- Johansson, S.G.O., Bennich, H. and Berg, T. (1972). The clinical significance of IgE. *Progr. Clin. Immunol.* 1 : 157-181.
- Kern, R. A. (1921). Dust sensitization in bronchial asthma. *Med Clin. North Am.* 5 : 751-758.

- Kjellman, N.I.M. (1977). Atopic disease in seven year old children. *Acta. Paediatr. Scand.* 66 : 465-471.
- Kumar, N. R., Kumar, R. and Singh, T. (1988). Faunistic and ecological studies on the Acaro-fauna of habitation of the socio-economically poor dwellers of Punjab and Himachal Pradesh, India. *Progress in Acarology* I:169-172.
- Kumud, R., Mathus, B. and Mathus, S. (1988). A preliminary report on the occurrence of house dust mites from Hisar, the subtropical region of Haryana, India. *Progress in Acarology* I:157-162.
- Lal, M. A., Dasgupta, A., Pande, J. N., Nayar, E. and Guleria, J. S.(1973). Clinical significance of skin reactions to mite extracts in individuals with bronchial asthma. *Ind. J. Med. Res.* 61 : 672-675.
- Matsumoto, K., Okamoto, M. and Wada, Y. (1986). Effects of relative humidity on life cycle of the house dust mites, *D. farinae* and *D. pteronyssinus. Jap. J. Sanit. Zool.*, 37: 79-90.
- Maurya, K. R., Dev, B. and Jamil, Z. (1983). Mites, insects and fungi associated with house dust from some regions of India (Abst.). Second *All India Sym. Acar.* Bangalore, p. 45.
- Modak, A., Saha, G. K., Gupta S. K. and Tandon, N. (1995). Occurrence of some uncommon dust mites from houses of respiratory allergic patients in West Bengal. *J. Acarol.* 13 (1&2) : 29-34.
- Modak, A., Saha, G. K., Tandon, N. and Gupta, S. K. (1991). Dust mite fauna in houses of bronchial asthma patients-comparative study of three zones of West Bengal, India. *Entomon* 16 (7) : 115-120.
- Modak A., Tandon, N. and Saha. G. K. (2000). Laboratory observation on the life cycle of *Dermatophagoides pteronyssinus* (Acarina, Pyroglyphidae) A common allergic mite of house dust. *Proc. Zool. Soc.* 53(2) : 105-108.
- Nayar, E., Lal, M. and Dasgupta, A. (1974). The prevalence of *D. pteronyssinus* and its association with house dust allergy. *Ind. J. Med. Res.* 62(1) : 11-14.
- Otani, T., Kinugawa, N., Likura, Y. and Hosjhi, F. (1984). Distribution of house-dust mites in the houses of asthmatic children in Japan. *Allergy Japan* (*Aerugi*) 33(8) : 454-462.
- Pepys, J., Chan, M. and Hargreave, F. E. (1968). Mites and house dust allergy. *Lancet* 1 : 1270-1272.
- Roy, S., Sharma, A., Chetty, A. and Sundaram, K. B. (1987). Skin test and RAST in children allergic to common allergens, *Ind. J. Pediatr.* 54: 437-440.
- Krishna Rao, N. S., Khuddus, C. A. and Channa Basavanna, G. P. (1973). Pyroglyphid mites in man and his surroundings. *Curr. Sci.* 42 : 33.
- Krishna Rao, N. S., Ranganath, H. R. and Channa Basavanna, G. P. (1981). House dust mites from India. *Indian J. Acar.* 5 : 85-94.

- Saha, G. K. (1993). House dust mite allergy in Calcutta, India: Evaluation by RAST. *Ann. Allergy* 70 : 305-309.
- Saha, G. K. (1994). Relationship between *Dermatophagoides* mite density and specific immune response in asthmatic patients. *Ann Allergy* 73 : 429-433.
- Saha, G.K. (1997) House dust mite sensitivity among rural and urban asthmatics of West Bengal, India : A comparison. *Aerobiologia* 13 : 269-273.
- Saha, G. K., Modak, A., Batabyal, S. K. Choudhuri, D. K., Maitra, S. B. and Tandon, N. (1989). Clinical significance of IgE in bronchial asthma. *J. Indian Med. Assoc.* 87(7) : 155-158.
- Saha, G. K., Modak, A., Tandon, N. and Choudhuri, D. K. (1995). The evaluation of skin prick test in house dust mite allergy in Calcutta, India. *Tropical and Geographical Medicine* 47(6) : 278-281.
- Shivpuri, D. N. (1981). House dust mite allergy in India. *Aspects of Allergy and Applied Immunology,* 14 : 19-35.
- Shivpuri, D. N. and Agarwal, M. K. (1971). Common precipitating causes of attacks of bronchial asthma in 174 patients. *Proceedings of the 26th National Conference on Tuberculosis and Chest Diseases,* p. 382.
- Spieksma, F. Th. M. (1967). Occurrence and properties of the house dust mite *Dermatophagoides pteronyssinus. Int. Rhinology* 5 : 162-167.
- Spieksma, F. Th. M., Zuidema, P. and Leupen, M. J. (1971). High altitude and house dust mites. *Br. Med. J.* 1 : 82-84.
- Tandon, N., Saha, G. K., Modak, A., Maitra, S. B., Kundu, S. C. and Batabayal, S. K. (1988). Mites in house dust as a cause of bronchial asthma. *J. Assoc. Physicians India* 36(2) : 141-144.
- Tandon, N., Maitra, S. B., Saha, G. K., Modak, A. and Hati, A. K. (1990). Role of cockroaches in allergy to house dust in Calcutta, India. *Ann. Allergy* 64 : 155-157.
- Tripathi, D. M. and Parikh, K. M. (1983). Mite fauna and other allergens present in the house dust in Bombay. *Lung India* 1(4): 147-151.
- Voorhorst, R. and Spieksma, F. Th. M. (1973). House dust atopy and the house dust mite *Dermatophagoides. Allergologia et Immunopathologia* 1(1) : 13-24.
- Voorhorst, R., Spieksma-Boezeman, M.I.A. and Spieksma, F. Th. M. (1964). Is a mite (*Dermatophagoides* sp.) the producer of house dust allergen? *Allergy Asthma* 10 : 329-334.
- Wharton, G. W. (1976). House dust mites. *J. Med. Entomol.* 12 : 577-621.
- Zheltikova, T. M., Petrova-Nikitina, A. D., Kanchurin, A. Kh., Berzhets, V. M. and Muzyleva, I. L. (1985). House dust mites and allergies in man. *Nauchyne Doklady Vysshei Shkoly, Biologicheskie Nauki,* 2 : 12-30.

Chapter - 12

Leishmaniasis

** Arnab Roy Chowdhury and Hemanta K Majumder**

Summary

Leishmaniasis has been, and still is one of the most major health problems afflicting millions of people worldwide. About thirty two different species or sub species of *Leishmania* are separately responsible for a complex set of deadly clinical symptoms. Lack of effective vaccines has made chemotherapy the only choice for combating this menace. Moreover, several present day drugs have limited efficacy due to high toxicity and the development of drug resistance. These have led to the search for new anti leishmanial agents having novel therapeutic targets. DNA topoisomerase(s) that catalyzes a variety of vital cellular processes have emerged as one such principal therapeutic target and promises to be the future.

Leishmaniasis

Leishmaniasis is one of the major health problems that at present has assumed a global dimension, and wrecks havoc in the tropical and subtropical countries. *Leishmania* are a group of unicellular protozoan parasites that are exclusively transmitted by the bite of female *Phlebotomus* sand flies. There are about 20 species of *Leishmania* parasites that are pathogenic to human. There is no absolute correlation between the *Leishmania* taxa and the clinical diseases produced, thereby making the actual detection of the disease and its treatment more difficult. To tackle this world wide threat to public health, the World Health Organization (WHO) in the year 1976 included leishmaniasis as one of the priority items in the UNDP/World Bank/WHO Special programme for research and training in tropical diseases (Peters and Killick-Kendrick,

* Molecular Parasistology Lab. Indian Institute of Chemical Biology, Kolkata

1987), along with the other major tropical diseases like malaria, filaria, trypanosomasis, leprosy and schistosomasis. Epidemiological data shows that leishmaniasis at present is the most fatal disease second only to malaria (WHO Chronicle, 1977). WHO reports indicate that about 6,00,000 new clinical cases of leishmaniasis are reported every year, with an overall prevalence of 12 million cases and an estimated population of 35 million being at risk (Desjeux, 1992). Therefore, the control and eradication of the disease has been one of the thrust areas identified by WHO and various scientists the world over are relentlessly fighting against this killer disease.

Geographic distribution

This distribution of *Leishmania* parasites primarily depend on the availability of vector flies as well as animal reservoirs. However, the parasites have a distribution almost through out the world, excepting for Australian and Antarctic continents. The prime endemic regions have been identified. A brief overview of the various *Leishmania* species, their geographic distribution, and the clinical pattern of the disease caused are presented in the table below.

Diseases Caused by *Leishmania* Species and their Geographic Distributions

Major species	Subspecies	Disease name	Clinical name	Distribution	Geo. occurrence
L.donovani	*L.d. donovani*	Kala-azar	VL,	Old world	Asia, Mediterranean basin,
	L.d. infantum		PKDL	Old world	Africa, South America
	L.d. chagasi			New world	
L. major		Oriental	CL	Old world	Central and South America,
		sore		New world	Southern Europe, Africa, Asia, Middle east, Southern Russia
L.tropica		Oriental	CL	Old world	Central and South America,
		sore	LR	New world	Southern Europe, Africa, Asia, Middle east
L.aethiopica		Oriental sore		Old world	Ethiopian highland, Mount Elgan in Kenya, South Yemen
L. mexicana	*L.m. mexicana* *L.m.amazonensis*	Chiclero's ulcer	CL DCL	New world	Mexico, Guatemala, Ama zon basin, Venazuela, Belize, Brazil and Trinidad Amazon basin
L.peruviana		Oriental sore	CL	New world	Western Peru
L braziliensis	*L.b. braziliensis*	Espundia	MCL	New world	South America
	L.b. guyanensis	Espundia	CL	New world	South America
	L.b. panamensis				

The Indian perspective: Kala-azar, or visceral leishmaniasis, is a major health concern in India. During 1991, it caused a large scale epidemic, and survey reports of six states show some 2.5 million visceral leishmaniasis cases, of which about 75,000 people died. In Bihar alone, 44 million people in 28 districts and about 5.5 million people in West Bengal are at risk of Kala-azar (WHO, 1993). According to official reports in the year 1992, leishmaniasis has spread further to the states of Uttar Pradesh and Orissa affecting about 80,000 people. Kala-azar is also reported from Tamilnadu in southern India and to a lesser extent from Delhi, Meghalaya and Pondicherry (Shanmugam *et al.*, 1977).

Clinical manifestations of different disease forms: Leishmaniasis is a common name given to at least three distinct diseases in human caused by a group of closely related protozoa. They are namely Visceral Leishmaniasis (VL), Cutaneous Leishmaniasis (CL) and Mucocutaneous Leishmaniasis (MCL) (Hoogstraal, *et al.*, 1967). The clinical features of the disease form can be elaborated as follows.

Visceral leishmaniasis (VL): The causative agents for this disease are *L. donovani donovani* in India, Africa (Naik, 1979; 1981), *L. donovani infantum* in the Mediterranean (Rocha, 1982) and *L. donovani chagasi* in South America (Napier *et al.*, 1930). Shortly after infection, the organisms are disseminated throughout the body and are taken up by the phagocytic cells in the lymph nodes, liver, spleen and bone marrow. The primary symptom is intermittent fever accompanied by cough and diarrhea. After a period lasting from a few weeks to several months, the characteristic illness referred to as Kala-azar develops. The abdomen gets distended due to massively enlarged liver and spleen (hepatosplenomegaly), causing abdominal discomforts. The disease is often fatal, with 100% mortality if untreated.

Post kala-azar dermal leishmaniasis (PKDL): It is a manifestation of visceral leishmaniasis following its apparent cure, and it is quite common among Indian patients. It often develops several years after the treatment of the acute disease. It is characterized by appearance of depigmented patches on skin, which progress to diffuse as nodular or papular lesions over the body. They are especially on the face, upper trunk, thighs, fore arms and legs. These hypopigmented macules and lesions may persist for several years after parasitological cure. The reappearance of parasites after apparent cure suggests that they might have survived within the host and stayed dormant. The PKDL patients are of considerable epidemiological importance (Napier, 1946).

Cutaneous leishmaniasis (CL): The species causing Old world cutaneous leishmaniasis include *L. major, L. tropica* and *L. aethiopiea. L. braziliensis* complexes cause the New World cutaneous leishmaniasis. It is a serious health problem in both Old and New world countries. The invading promastigotes adapt to amastigotes life form in skin macrophages and this in turn elicits a host immune response. A crust of epithelial cells and dried inflammatry cells frequently covers the ulcer of cutaneous leishmaniasis. Chronicity is the feature of the cutaneous infection. Poor response to treatment is more characteristic of *L. braziliensis braziliensis* infections. Lesions that develop in the pinna of the ear are associated with a protracted course of tissue destruction, the so called "Chiclero's Ulcer".

Diffuse cutaneous leishmanisis (DCL): In the Old world, DCL is associated with *L. aethiopica,* where as in America, *L. mexicana* and *L. amazonesis* has been ascertained as the responsible factors. It is recognized that DCL is manifested only in patients with an abnormal immune response and that the same parasite would normally cause ulcerating simple lesions in the general population (Convit *et al.* 1971). The defining features of this disease entity is formation of lesions that are non- ulcerating nodules and plaques representing lepromatous leprosy. The condition is almost refractory to chemotherapy.

Mucocutaneous leishmaniasis (MCL): Mucocutaneous leishmaniasis or Espundia, is best known for its dramatic mutilating lesions. It is caused primarily by *L. braziliensis braziliensis,* and is a major health problem in Central America (Pessoa *et al.,* 1944). Prolonged incubation causes the degradation and necrosis of the mucous layer. When early and effective treatment is not available even the least serious form of the leishmaniasis, can lead to a serious problem like permanent facial mutilation for the victim.

Leishmania *recividans*(LR): It is a hypersensitive dermal response primarily associated with a chronic recurrence of *L. tropica* in the Middle East. The disease is marked by the appearance of nodular lesions and satellite lesions at margins of healed primary lesions. Like DCL, the disease is not easily cured.

Leishmania/ *HIV co infections:* The global scenario becomes further grim due to the rapid spread of Human Immunodeficiency Virus (HIV). It provides additional scope to leishmaniasis, which thrives as an oppurtunistic infection (Fuzibet *et al.,* 1988; Ashford *et al.,* 1992). According to WHO the Leishmania/HIV co infection should be included among the AIDS defining diseases. The proposed definition of leishmaniasis as an AIDS defining disease is: "Any patient with co existing HIV infection and visceral leishmaniasis". It was reported that in Southern Europe *Leishmania*/HIV co infection occurred in severely immunosuppressed patients, and there is quick evolution from infection to disease. There are also reports of frequent, severe, visceral leishmaniasis in HIV positive patients caused by the *Leishmania* strains that are of low or no virulence in HIV negative individuals. During co infention, multiple visceral localization outside the reticulo-endothelial system are frequent viz. in the blood, normal skin, gastro-intestinal tract, lungs and central nervous system. The frequency of *Leishmania* in the peripheral blood is increased noticeably. This in turn enhances the chances of disease transmission through sand fly bites.

General biology of *Leishmania* parasites

Systematic classification: The systematic position of the pathogenic protozoan *Leishmania* is as follows:

KINGDOM	:	Protista
PHYLUM	:	Protozoa
SUBPHYLUM	:	Sarcomastigophora
SUPERCLASS	:	Mastigophora
CLASS	:	Zoomastigophora
ORDER	:	Kinetoplastida
SUBORDER	:	Trypanosomatina
FAMILY	:	Trypanosomatidae
GENUS	:	*Leishmania*

Morphology: *Leishmania* exists in two stages:

Amastigote stage: The amastigote or aflagellar stage occurs in vertebrate hosts with the parasite residing in the cells of reticulo-endothelial system of man, dog and hamsters. The parasite is round or oval shaped, 2-4μm long, along the longitudinal axis with little or no motility. Although the cellular organelles are similar to the promastigote form, in place of flagellum there is a delicate filament extending from the basal body to the margin of the body, which represents the root of the flagellum in the amastigote.

Promastigote stage: The promastigote is the extracellular form of the parasite only detected in cultures or in insect vectors. Fully developed promastigotes have long, slender spindle-shaped body measuring 15-20μm in length. The nucleus is situated centrally and the kinetoplast lies transversely near anterior end. The flagellum may be of the same length as the body or even longer, projecting from the front.

Life-cycle: *Leishmania* species have a dimorphic life cycle alternating between humans, as primary reservoirs, and sand flies, as secondary hosts. Metacyclic promastigotes are transferred to the vertebrate host from the sand fly as the latter takes a blood meal. Within the vertebrate hosts the promastigotes are phagocytosed by the macrophages, which then fuse with the lysosomes. The acidic pH and the hydrolytic enzymes within the lysosome are unable to destroy the parasites as they are resistant to them. Moreover, the parasites shut down the generation of the reactive oxygen intermediates by the macrophage and effectively convert to an amastigote. These amastigotes replicate by binary fission and fill up the macrophage. Finally amastigotes are released from the infected macrophage and re-initiate this replicative cycle in new macrophages. Ingestion of infected macrophages by sand flies results in the conversion of amastigotes to promastigotes, which replicate by binary fission and adhere to the gut epithelium of sand fly to avoid being excreted. The procyclic promastigotes then quit dividing and undergoes a terminal differentiation into metacyclic promastigotes which are infective for the vertebrate hosts (Chang *et al.*, 1985).

Immunobiology of leishmaniasis: During Kala-azar, the cell mediated immunity and delayed hypersensitivity reaction of the skin to *Leishmania* antigen does not develop until the disease has been cured. This is because *L. donovani* infection induces immunesuppressive effect and as a result there is no host response. Hence, the cells of the reticulo-endothelia of the affected organs proliferate and become heavily parasitized. In contrast, during *L. tropica* infection, a well-marked cell mediated immunity appears early accompanied by the development of a delayed hypersensitivity reaction and elimination of parasites. Two conditions in which cell mediated immunity remains ineffective in clearing cutaneous parasites are leishmaniasis recivida and leishmaniasis tegumentaria diffusa.

Diagnosis of leishmaniasis: Diagnosis of *L. donovani* depends on finding amastigotes in tissues or secretions. Spleen punctures, blood or nasal smears, bone marrow and other tissues are examined for the characteristic parasites. Immunodiagnostic tools are sensitive but cannot differentiate between species of *Leishmania* and between current and cured cases. The tests most frequently used are the enzyme-linked immunosorbent assay (ELISA) and the indirect fluorescence antibody test. Until recently, the main limitations of these tests were a cross reacting positive response to

Trypanosoma cruzi. This problem has been resolved by improved techniques of antigen purification, special antigen polymerization and antigen selection by use of monoclonal antibodies. Recently, PCR based diagnosis by genus specific (Bhattacharya *et al.*, 1996) and species specific primers (Rogers *et al.*, 1990; Bhattacharya *et al.*, 1993) have also been developed as a tool for diagnosis. Other diseases that might have symptoms similar to kala-azar are typhoid and paratyphoid fevers, malaria, syphilis, tuberculosis, dysentery and relapsing fevers. Each must be eliminated in the diagnosis of Kala-azar.

Chemotherapy against leishmaniasis

Leishmaniasis, one of the most dreaded diseases threatening mankind, does not have enough combative measures. Development of vaccines is still far from reality, though research and trial programmes are continuing. Therefore, chemotherapy remains the only practical means of combating the disease. Ehlrich and his associates in Germany towards the end of the last century developed chemotherapy as a means of controlling infectious diseases. Their rationale of achieving drug selectively through differential toxicity towards host and pathogen still remains as the basis to all modern day drug development. Several of the antileishmanial drugs show serious side effects in the host, and thus are not suitable for long-term treatment measure. Although pentavalent antimonials still remain the mainstay of treatment against leishmaniasis, the compounds are highly toxic. Therefore improved drug therapy is still desirable and is a demanding challenge in the field of modern pharmaceutical research.

Present scenario: The present scene has been gloomy, as over the years it has been evidenced that protozoan parasites have become unresponsive to antimonials. A recent finding that *L. tropica* is coendemic agent of visceral leishmaniasis in India (Sacks *et al.*, 1995), explains the rising frequency of unresponsiveness to sodium antimony gluconate therapy, which complicates the treatment in Indian subcontinent. Pentamidine and amphotericin B have been prescribed by WHO as second-line drug for the treatment of unresponsive or relapse cases of visceral leishmaniasis (WHO, 1995). The high cure rate achieved by amphotericin B has resulted in its use to treat large number of multidrug-resistant kala-azar patients. However, the drug being quite expensive is yet to find a greater use. Pyrazolopyrimidines and 8-aminoquinolines have also shown significant promise. Of these compounds, allopurinol (4 hydroxy pyrazole [3,4-d] pyrimidine), a structural analogue of hypoxanthine, interferes with the purine metabolism and is effective against *L. donovani* and *L. mexicana* (Kager *et al.*, 1981). One lepidine compound, WR6026 belonging to the 8-aminoquinoline class, is another potential chemotherapeutic agent against leishmaniasis (Berman, 1985). Other compounds with notable antileishmanial effect are hamycin (Banerjee *et al.*, 1994; Sarkar *et al.*, 1992) a polyene antibiotic, and doxorubicin (Di Macro *et al.*, 1975; Zunino and Capranico, 1990), an anthracycline antibiotic. To reduce the toxic side effects of these drugs, liposome encapsulation has been found to be very effective (Chance, 1980; Robinovitch and Altieri, 1987). The search for an efficacious, less toxic yet inexpensive drug is the requirement of the day to fight against leishmaniasis.

Natural compounds: Studies of plant derived natural compounds, as candidate chemotherapeutic agents are a fast emerging field. More than 20 plant species belonging to various taxonomic groups contain compounds that show promising antileishmanial activity. These compounds belong to diverse chemical groups, namely, benzylisoquinolines, â-carbonyl alkaloids, iridoid and steroidal glycosides, quinones and quinolones (Iwu *et al.*, 1994). Development of these indigenous plant derived products into potent antileishmanial drugs may open up a new avenue to combat this protozoan disease.

Newer drugs and approaches: Preliminary results are promising for other drugs and therapeutic approaches that are currently being studied, but clinical experience is not adequate to justify their general use. The types of drugs under investigation include cytokines such as interferon gamma (IFG) and granulocyte macrophage colony-stimulating factor (GM-CSF) (both used in combination of pentavalent antimony) (Ho *et al.*, 1994; Badaro *et al.*, 1990; Harms *et al.*, 1991); aminoglycosides such as paromomycin (used as monotherapy or with pentavalent antimony) (Berman, 1997); oral antifungal agents such as ketokonazole (monotherapy) (Berman, 1996) an allopurinol (used with pentavalent antimony) (Martinez *et al.*, 1997). Local treatment of CL, such as intralesional antimony (Faris *et al.*, 1993) and topical paromomycin (15%) plus methylbenzethonium chloride (12%) in combination with antimony injections have also been studied (Berman, 1996). Another drug for future is hexadecylphosphocholine or miltefosine, a phospholipid derivative which was basically developed as an anti tumour agent. WHO sponsored trials are on after which it could be formally registered for the treatment of kala-azar (Sundar *et al.*, 1998).

First vaccine trial against visceral leishmaniasis: The results of the first trial of a vaccine against visceral leishmaniasis in humans have been published in The Lancet by Khalil *et al.* (2000). In a study performed by scientists of the Institute of Endemic Diseases, a vaccine composed of autoclaved *Leishmania major* promastigotes mixed with a low dose of BCG (as adjuvant) was compared with BCG alone. The *Leishmania* + BCG vaccine did induce significantly higher rates of Leishmanin skin test (LST) conversion (30% vs. 7% by BCG alone) at 42 days which was associated with lower incidence of disease. However, there is a need to identify a suitable adjuvant to improve immunogenicity of killed *Leishmania* vaccines. Recent preliminary studies in Sudan are highly encouraging since various doses induced a strong LST conversion in all volunteers.

Unique Feature of trypanosomatid protozoa : kinetoplast DNA

The first report of kinetoplast containing genetic material goes way back to 1898, when Ziemann reported that the organelle stained a brilliant red similar to the nucleus (Shapiro and Englund, 1995). Later stages show the emergence of kinetoplast DNA (kDNA) as one of the most unusual features of the trypanosomatid protozoa. The kDNA, unique in its structure, function and mode of replication, is actually a giant DNA network (10^{10} kDa) consisting of several thousand circular DNAs that are topologically interlocked. Each cell contains one network condensed into a disk-shaped structure within the matrix of its single mitochondrion. This magnificently intriguing molecular configuration of kDNA was revealed by electron microscopic studies in the later 1960s and early 1970s (Laurent *et al.*, 1970; Riou *et al.*, 1969). The isolated network has an elliptical shape about 10-15 μm with a fairly regular structure. The network contains two types of DNA molecules: maxicircles present in a few dozen copies and minicircles present in a few thousand copies. The maxicircles, which encode ribosomal RNAs and a few mitochondrial proteins are similar in structure and function to the mitochondrial DNA of other eukaryotes. Minicircles, on the other hand, encode small guide RNAs which control the specificity of editing, but till date there is no report of minicircle encoded protein.

The molecular components of kDNA:

Maxicircles: Maxicircles are nothing but the functional homologues of mitochondrial DNA in other eukaryotes. Their size varies from species to species, in the range of 20-40 kb. Maxicircles encode ribosomal RNAs and several proteins, most of which are involved in mitochondrial energy transduction (e.g., cytochrome b, subunits of cytochrome oxidase and subunits of NADH dehydrogenase). However, they apparently do not encode tRNAs. A most remarkable feature of the maxicircle is that most of their transcripts undergo RNA editing to form a functional mRNA (Benne *et al.,* 1986). RNA editing is the process of addition or detection of uridine residues at specific sites in the transcript, and in some mRNAs more than half of the nucleotides in the coding sequence are introduced by editing (Feagin *et al.,* 1988).

Minicircles : Minicircles makes up over 90% of the mass of the kDNA network with 5 X 10^3 - 10^4 copies per network. They vary in size from species to species within a range of 0.5 to 2.9 kb. In most species, all the minicircles in a network are about the same size, e.g., in *Leishmania* they are about 830 bp. Minicircles perform crucial genetic function of encoding small guide RNAs, about 70 nucleotides long with a short non-encoded oligo-U tail at *3'-end,* that govern the specificity of RNA editing (Sturm *et al.,* 1990). In most kinetoplastids including *Leishmania,* the minicircle sequences are heterogeneous which is a reflection of the wide number of guide RNAs required for editing. *Trypanosoma brucei,* for example, contains over 250 different minicircle sequence classes, all differing in copy number (Steinert *et al.,* 1980). In *L. donovani,* minicircle sequences can be classified into major and minor class (Singh *et al.,* 1994). Again, both these classes consist of minicircles of different sequences. However, in *Crithidia fasciculata,* 90% of the minicircles have about the same sequence (Sugisaki *et al.,* 1987).

In spite of this apparent heterogeneity in the minicircle sequences, they also possess conserved sequence regions (usually 100 - 180 nucleotides), that are virtually identical in all minicircles. The minicircle replication origin lies within this region. Some minicircles, like those in *L. donovani, L. tarentolae,* and *T. brucei* (Singh *et al.,* 1994) contain a single conserved region, whereas *C. fasciculata* minicircles contain two (Sugisaki *et al.,*1987) conserved regions. Multiple conserved regions, when present, are usually positioned 180^0 or 90^0 apart on the minicircle map.

DNA topoisomerases - the wonder enzymes

The various problems of disentangling DNA strands or duplexes in a cell are rooted in the double helical structure of DNA. DNA topoisomerases are the distinct family of enzymes that have evolved to solve these problems. Topoisomerases probably entered the stage of evolution when the increasing length of DNA or the formation of duplex rings created topological problems that needed to be resolved for propagation of the genetic material. The topological problems are, for example, unraveling of the complimentary DNA strands during replication, disentanglement of duplex DNA molecules during chromosomal condensation and segregation etc. DNA topoisomerases catalyze the passage of individual DNA strands or double helices through one another and these reactions are often manifested in interconversion between topological isomers of DNA rings and hence the name of the enzymes.

Classes of DNA topoisomerases : In spite of their functional and genetic distinctiveness, DNA topoisomerases are broadly classified into two types; (i) type I, whose reactions involve transient single stranded breakage in absence of any high energy co-factor and (ii) type II, whose reactions involve formation of transient double stranded breaks in the presence of ATP. Type I topoisomerases change the linking number in steps of one whereas type II enzymes change the linking number in steps of II (Brown and Cozzarelli, 1979; Liu *et al.*, 1989). However, the basic mechanistic steps involved in the reactions catalyzed by both types of topoisomerases are two successive trans-esterification reactions. In the first reaction, the tyrosine hydroxyl group from enzyme active site attacks a DNA phosphodiester bond. As a result the enzyme becomes linked to a 5' - phosphoryl group (3'-phosphoryl group for eukaryotic DNA topoisomerase I) with a free deoxyribose hydroxyl group. The second reaction sees the nucleophilic attack of the phospho-tyrosine linkage by the deoxyribose hydroxyl group, which rejoins the DNA strand and frees the enzyme from covalent attachment to the DNA. Therefore, a topoisomerase reaction can be summarized in four steps i) DNA binding ii) cleavage of one or both DNA strands iii) passage of a segment of DNA through this break, and iv) resealing of the DNA break.

Type I DNA topoisomerase : The main reaction catalyzed by topoisomerase I is the relaxation of supercoiled DNA (Gellert, 1981). However, bacterial topoisomerase I cannot relax positively supercoiled DNA unlike its mammalian counterparts (Wang, 1985). Apart from the relaxation of positively and negatively supercoiled DNA, topoisomerase I also perform the following functions : i) knotting and unknotting of single stranded DNA rings (Liu, 1976) ii) intertwining of covalently closed single stranded DNA rings with complimentary base sequences (Kirkegaard and Wang, 1978) and iii) catenation and decatenation of single stranded DNA rings, one of which is nicked (Low *et al.*, 1984).

***Type II DNA topoisomerase*:** Type II topoisomerases introduce a transient break into the double strand of DNA backbone so as to create an enzyme operated gate, through which the complimentary strand is allowed to pass via a energy requiring mechanism (Voseberg, 1985). The three basic reactions catalyzed by topoisomerase II are as follows : i) relaxation or supercoiling of covalently closed circular DNA ii) knotting or unknotting of double stranded DNA rings and iii) catenation or decatenation of double stranded DNA rings (Maxwell and Gellart, 1986). Within this subgroup, only bacterial gyrase can catalÿze negative supercoiling, whereas the other members, in spite of their ATP requirement, can relax negatively or positively supercoiled DNA, but not the reverse action (Liu, 1994).

Biological functions of topoisomerases : "cell magicians"

As enzymes DNA topoisomerases are magicians of the cell; they open and close gates within a DNA without leaving a trace. Since their biological functions are deeply rooted in the double helix structure of DNA, it is not surprising that these enzymes participate in nearly all biological processes involving DNA. They are involved in replication, transcription, recombination, maintenance of chromosome structure and genomic stability, chromosomal condensation and chromosomal segregation (Liu, 1994).

Topoisomerases as therapeutic targets :

Current biomedical research has its focus on the search for newer intervention strategies to control the public health impact of parasitic diseases. The dramatic advances of molecular and cellular biology in recent times have provided opportunities for discovering and evaluating molecular targets for drug designing, which now form a rational basis for the development of improved antiparasitic therapy.

Drug targets in kinetoplastid parasites, exemplified by cysteine proteases and trypanothione reductase, have been purified and used for inhibitor screening (Werbovetz, 2000). Other findings show that successful antifolate chemotherapy in *Leishmania* will have to target simultaneously both dihydrofolate reductase (DHFR) and pteridine reductase (PTR - 1) (Nare *et al.*, 1990). Studies show that the parasite topoisomerases are sufficiently distinct from their human counterparts so as to allow differential chemical targeting and will therefore make good target for antiparasitic drug discovery.

Despite differences in cataytic mechanisms and cellular functions, the critical feature common to all topoisomerases is the DNA cleavage and subsequent strand passage event. Under normal conditions, the covalent enzyme DNA cleavable complexes are fleeting catalytic intermediates and are present in low steady state concentrations. Consequently, the cell tolerates them. However, conditions that significantly decrease or increase the physiological concentrations of these breaks unleash a myriad of deleterious side effects, including mutations, insertions, deletions and chromosomal aberrations (Stacie *et al.*, 1995). Thus, all topoisomerases are fundamentally dualistic in nature; catalyzing essential cellular reactions and possessing an inherent dark side capable of inflicting great harm to the genome of an organism.

In lieu of this, science of DNA topoisomerases have evolved from basic DNA enzymology to targeted therapeutics and topoisomerases have been recognized as potential chemotherapeutic targets for anti tumor and anti parasitic agents (Liu, 1989; Chakraborty *et al.*, 1988; D' Arpa and Liu, 1989; Drlica and Franco, 1988).

Topoisomerase inhibitors : The known DNA topoisomerase inhibitors can be divided into two classes, i) class I inhibitors and ii) class II inhibitors. The class I drugs act by stabilizing the covalent topoisomerase-DNA complexes and are also referred to as " topoisomerase poisons" (Kreuzer and Cozarelli, 1979). They include the bacterial gyrase quinoline antibiotics, the DNA topoisomerase I inhibitor camptothecin and the DNA topoisomerase II inhibitors doxorubicin, amsacrine, etoposide teniposide, quercetin and related flavonoids (Kreuzer and Cozarelli, 1979; Liu, 1989; Drlica and Franco, 1988).

The stabilization of cleavable complexes by these class I poisons subsequently leads to cell death, but the process leading to it is a myriad of complex pathways, namely, (i) initiation of damage induced signaling (ii) cell cycle alterations with subsequent arrest and (iii) engagement of enzymatic machinery that results in apoptosis. However, a fraction of the cells treated with topoisomerase poisons survive the treatment due to DNA repair mechanisms. Nonetheless, they contain an increased frequency of chromosomal aberrations and mutations. Programmed cell death after treatment of topoisomerase directed agents are brought about by i) stress activated kinases and death receptor pathways and ii) caspase activation resulting to caspase mediated cleavages (Kaufmann, 1988).

The class II drugs interfere with the catalytic functions of DNA topoisomerases without trapping the covalent complexes, and they have been referred to as "catalytic inhibitors". These classes of drugs include the coumermycin family of antibiotics that act on bacterial gyrase (Drlica and Franco, 1988) and the eukaryotic topoisomerase II inhibitors suramin (Bojanowski *et al.*, 1992), fostriecin (Boritzki *et al.*, 1988), merbarone (Drake *et al.*, 1989) and bis 2, 6-dioxopiparazine (Tanabe *et al.*, 1991). Several inhibitors of eukaryotic topoisomerase I have also been reported (Burry *et al.*, 1992)..

All class II drugs mediate their action by either binding to the enzyme, which prevents it to sit on the substrate DNA, e.g. merbarone (Drake *et al.* 1989) and aceteyl boswellic acids (Syrovets *et al.* 2000) or by intercataling/binding to DNA and making it inaccessible for the enzyme, e.g. aclarubin and chloroquine. Coumermycins interact with gyrase ATPase domain and thus interfere with the ATPase activity (delCastillo *et al.*, 1991). DNA topoisomerases are truly wonder enzymes. The fact that they are targets for various chemotherapeutic agents has led to a rapid progress in understanding the dynamic nature of the enzymes in relation to the cell survival and in the development of new therapeutics. Important enzymens in the life cycle of the parasite are also being studied in different laboratories of the world, e.g. cysteine protease, trypanthione reductase, dihydro folate reductase etc. DNA topoisomerases have evolved as an important therapeutic target and is being extensively studied as of today. The screening of bioactive compounds and synthesis of selective topoisomerase inhibitors will help to develop better topoisomerase specific drugs for the future.

Leishmaniasis is the one of most fatal parasitic disease affecting millions around the world. Though there has been a tremendous progress in understanding the molecular biology of *Leishmania* in recent years, drug toxicity and resistance, with the absence of effective newer drugs; demand the discovery of novel therapeutic agents. Studies on DNA topoisomerases and the kDNA of the organism will be of great help in developing newer drugs to fight against this devastating disease.

Different classes of DNA topoisomerase inhibitors

Class of drugs	Topoisomerase inhibitors	Types of topoismerase
Quinolones	Nalidixic acid, Oxonolic acid, Piromidic acid	gyrase
Fluoroquinolones	Norfloxacin, Ciprofloxacin, Ofloxacin, Enoxacin	gyrase/topo II ?
Coumarins	Novobiocin, Coumermycin A1, Chlorobion	gyrase/topo II ?
Anthracyclins	Adriamycin, Doxorubicin, Daunorubicin	topo II & gyrase
Podophyllotoxins	Teniposide, Etoposide, Etophos, NK611	topo II
Alkaloids	Camptothecin, Topotecan, CPT-11, Nitidine.	topo I
MGDBs	Distamyscin, Hoechest 33342, Berenil, Netropsin	topo I
Acridines	m-AMSA, 9-anilino acridines	topo II
Ellipticines	2-Me 9-OH Et, Pazelliptine, Anatoxin, Datelliptium.	topo II
Antibiotics	Saintopin, Topostin, Stretonigrin	topo I & topo II
Benzophenazine	NC-190	topo II
Flavonoids	Genistein, Woodfructicosin	topo II
Terpenoids	terpenticin, Cleroxidin	topo II
Dioxopiperazine	Sobuzoxane, Razoxane, ICRF-154, ICRF-193	topo II
Indolocarbazole	ED-110, KT-6528	topo I
Makaluvamines	Makaluvamine derivatives	topo II
Antimonials	Sodium stibogluconate, Urea stibamine	*Leishmania* topo I
Lignanolides	(-)-Arctigenin, (-)-Trachelogenin	topo II

References

- Ashford, R.W., Kohestany, K.A. and Karinzad, M.A. (1992) Cutaneous leishmaniasis in Kabul: observations on 'prolonged epidemic'. *Ann. Trop. Med. Parasitol.* **86**, 361.
- Badaro, R. and Johnson, W.D. (1993) The role of interferon-gamma in the treatment of visceral and diffuse cutaneous leishmaniasis. *J. Infect. Dis.* **167** (suppl 1), S13.
- Banerjee, G., Bhaduri, A.N. and Basu, M.K. (1994) Mannose-coated liposomal hamycin in the treatment of experimental leishmaniasis in hamsters. *Biochem. Med. Biol. Chem.* **53**, 1.

- Beene, R., Van Den Burg, J., Brakenhoff, J.P.J., Sloof, P. and Van Bloom, J.H. (1986) Major transcript of the frame-shifted coxII gene from trypanosome mitochondria contains four nucleotides that are not encoded in the DNA. *Cell* **46**, 819.
- Berman, J.D. (1988) Chemotherapy for leishmaniasis: biochemical, mechanisms, clinical efficacy and strategies. *Rev. Infect. Dis.*, May-June; **10**(3), 560.
- Berman, J.D. (1996) Treatment of new world cutaneous and mucosal leishmaniasis. *Clin. Dermatol.* **14**, 519.
- Berman, J.D. (1997) Human leishmaniasis: clinical, diagnostic and chemotherapeutic developments in the last 10 years. *Clin. Infect. Dis.* **24**, 684.
- Berry, D.E. Naturally occurring inhibitors of topoisomerase I mediated DNA relaxation. *J. Org. Chem.* **57**, 420.
- Bettini, S., Maroli, M., Gradoni, L. (1981) Leishmaniasis in Tuscany (Italy): (IV) An analysis of all recorded human cases. *Trans. R. Soc. Trop. Med. Hyg.* **75**(3), 338.
- Bhattacharya, R., Singh, R., Hazra, T.K. and **Majumder, H.K.** (1993) Application of polymerase chain reaction with specific and arbitrary primers to identification and differentiation of Leishmania parasites. *FEMS Microbiol Lett.* **114**, 99.
- Bhattacharya, R., Das, K., Sen, S., Roy, S. and **Majumder, H.K.** (1996) Development of a genus specific primer set for detection of Leishmania parasites by polymerase chain reaction. *FEMS Microbiol Lett.* **135**, 195.
- Bojanowski, K., Lelievre, S., Markovits, J., Coupne, J., Jacquemin-Sablon, A. and Larsen, A.K. (1992) Suramin is an inhibitor of DNA topoisomerase II in vitro and in Chinese hamster fibrosarcoma cells. *Proc. Natl. Acad. Sci.* USA **89**, 3025.
- Boritzki, J.T., Wolfard, S.T., Besserper, J.A., Jackson, R.C. and Fry, D.W. (1988) Inhibition of type II topoisomerase by fostriecin. *Biochem. Pharmacol.* **37**, 4063.
- Brown, P.O. and Cozarelli, R. (1979) A sign inversion mechanism for enzymatic supercoiling of DNA. *Science* **206**, 1081.
- Chakraborty, A.K. and **Majumder, H.K.** (1988) Mode of action of pentavalent antimonials: Specific inhibition of type I DNA topoisomerase of Leishmania donovani. *Biochem. Biophys. Res. Commun.* **152**, 605.
- Chance, M.L. (1980) In: Liposomes in Biological System (Gregoriadis, G. and Allison, A.C. eds.) Willey and Sons, New York.
- Chang, K.P., Fang, D., Bray, R.S. (1985) Biology of Leishmania and leishmaniasis. In: Leishmaniasis, Chang, K.P. and Bray, R.S. (eds.) Elsevier Biomedical Press, Amsterdam.

- Convit, J., Pinard, M.E., Rondon, A.J. (1972) Diffuse cutaneous leishmaniasis: a disease due to an immunological defect of the host. *Trans. R. Soc. Trop. Med. Hyg.* **66**(4), 603.
- DelCastillio, I., Vizan, J.L., Rodriquez-Sainz, M.C. and Moreno, F. (1991) An unusual mechanism for resistance to the antibiotic coumermycin A1. *Proc. Natl. Acad. Sci.* USA **88**, 8860.
- DiMacro, A., Acramone, R., Zunino, F. (1975) In: Antibiotics III: Mechanism of action of antimicrobial and antitumor agents (Corcoran, J.W. and Hahn, F.E. eds.) Springer-Verlag, New York.
- Drake, F.H., Hoffmann, G.A., Mong, S.M., Bartus, H.F., Hettzberg, R.P., Johnson, R.K., Mattern, M.R. and Mirabelli, C.K. (1989) In vitro and intracellular inhibition of topoisomerase II by the antitumor agent merbarone. *Cancer Res.* **49**, 2578.
- Falcoff E Taranto NJ, Remondegui CE, Debet JP, Canini L.M., Ripll CM, Dimier-David L., Vargas F., Gimenez LA and Bernabo, J.G. (1994) Clinical healing of antimony-resistant cutaneous or mucocutaneous leishmaniasis following the combined administration of interferongamma and pentavalent antimonial compounds. *Trans. R. Soc. Trop. Med. Hyg.* **88**, 95.
- Fari, R.M., Jarallah, J.S., Khoja, T.A. and Al-Yamani, M.J. (1993) Intralesional treatment of cutaneous leishmaniasis with sodium stibogluconate antimony. *Int. J. Dermatol.* **32**, 610.
- Feagin, J.E., Abraham, J.M. and Stuart, K. (1988) Characterization of cytochrome c oxidase III transcripts that are edited only in the 3′ region. *Cell* **53**, 413.
- Fuzibet, J.G., Marty, P., Taillan, B., Bertrand, F., Prof. P., Pesce, A., Le Fischoux, Y. and Dujardin, P. (1988) Is Leishmania infantum an opportunistic parasite in patients with anti-human immunodeficiency virus antibodies? *Arch. Intern Med.* **148**, 1228.
- Gellert, M. (1981) DNA topoisomerases. *Annu Rev. Biochem* **50**, 879.
- Harms, G., Chehade, A.K., Douba, M., Roepke, M., Mouakeh, A., Rosenkaimer, F. and Bienzle, U. (1991) A randomized trial comparing a pentavalent antimonial drug and recombinant interferon-gamma in the local treatment of cutaneous leishmaniasis. *Trans. R. Soc. Trop. Med. Hyg.* **85**, 214.
- Ho, J.L., Badaro, R., Hatzigeorgiou, D., Reed, S.G. and Johnson, W.D. Jr. (1994). Cytokines in the treatment of leishmaniasis: from studies of immunopathology to patient therapy. *Biotherapy* **7**, 223.
- Hoogstraal, H. and Heynemann, D. (1969) Leishmaniasis in the Sudan Republic 30, Final epidemiologic report. *Am. Soc. Trop. Hyg.* **83**, 119.
- Iwu, M.M., Jackson, J.E. and Schuster, B.G. (1994) Medicinal plants in the fight against leishmaniasis. *Parasitol. Today.* **10**, 65.

- Kager, P.A., Ree, P.H., Wellde, B.T., Hockmeyer, W.T., Lyerly W.H. (1981) Allopurinol in the treatment of visceral leishmaniasis. *Trans. Royal. Soc. Trop. Med. Hyg.* **77,** 204.
- Kaufmann, S.H. (1988) Cell death Induced by topoisomerase targeted drugs: more questions than answers. *Biochemica et Biophica Acta* **1400,** 195.
- Kirkegaard, K. and Wang, J.C. (1978) Escherichia coli DNA topoisomerase I catalyzed linking of single-stranded rings of complementary base sequences. *Nucleic Acids Res.* **5,** 3811.
- Kreuzer, K.N. and Cozarelli, N.R. (1980) Formation and resolution of DNA catenanes by DNA gyrase. *Cell* **20,** 245.
- Laurent, M. and Steinert, M. (1970) Electron microscopy of kinetoplastic DNA from Trypanosoma mega. *Proc. Natl. Acad. Sci.* USA **66,** 419.
- Liu, L.F., Depew, R.E. and Wang], J.C. (1976) Knotted single-stranded DNA rings: a novel topological isomer of circular single-stranded DNA formed by treatment with Escherichia coli omega protein *J. Mol. Bio.* **106,** 439.
- Liu, L.F., Liu, C.C. ad Alberts B.M. (1980) Type II DNA topoisomerases: enzymes that can unknot a topologically knotted DNA molecular via a reversible double-strand break. *Cell* **19,** 697.
- Liu, L.F. (1989) DNA topoisomerase poisons as antitumor drugs. *Annu. Rev. Biochem.* **58,** 351.
- Liu, L.F. (1994) DNA topoisomerases: Biochemistry and Molecular Biology. In: Advances in pharmacology, Vol. **29A**, Liu, L.F. (eds.) Academic Press, New York.
- Martinez, S., Gonzalez, M. and Vernaza, M.E. (1997) Treatment of cutaneous leishmaniasis with allopurinol and stibogluconate. *Clin. Infect. Dis.* **24,** 165.
- Mattern, M.R. and Mirabelli, C.K. (1989) In vitro and intracellular inhibition of topoisomerase II by the antitumor agent merbarone. *Cancer Res.* **49,** 2578.
- Maxwell, A. and Gellert, M. (1986) Mechanistic aspects of DNA topoisomerases. *Adv. Protein. Chem.* **38,** 69.
- Naik, S.R. (1979) Kala-azar in north-western India: a study of 24 patients. Trans. *R. Soc. Trop. Med. Hyg.* **73,** 61.
- Napier, L.E. and Dasgupta, C.R. (1930) *Ind. Med. Gazette* **65,** 249.
- Napier, L.E. (1946) The principal and Practice of Tropical Medicine, The MacMillan company: New York.
- Nare', B., Hardy, L.W. and Beverly, S.M. (1997) The roles of pteridine reductase 1 and dihydrofolate reductase-thymidylate synthase in pteridine metabolism in the protozoan parasite Leishmania major. *J. Biol. Chem.* **272,** 13883.

- Navin, T.R., Arana, F.E., de Merida, A.M., Arana, B.A., Castillo, A.L. and Silvers, D.N. (1992) Placebo-controlled clinical trial of sodium stibogluconate (Pentostam) versus ketoconazole for treating cutaneous leish, maniasis in Guatemale. *J. Infect. Dis.* **165**, 528.
- Peters, W. and Killick-Kendrick, R. (1987) In the preface of "The Leishmaniasis in Biology and Medicine", Vol **I**, Peters, W. Killick-Kendrick, R. (eds.) Academic Press, London.
- Pessoa, S.B. and Barreto, M.P. (1944) *Leishmaniose tegumentar Americana. Ministerio Da Educacao E. Saude, Servico de Documentacao.* Imprensa Nacional: Rio de Janerio, 527.
- Riou, G. and Delain, E. (1969) Abnormal circular DNA molecules induced by ethidium bromide in the kinetoplast of Trypanosama cruzi. *Proc. Natl. Acad. Sci.* USA **62**, 210.
- Rabinovitch, M., Alfieri, S.C. (1987) From lysosomes to cells, from cells to leishmania: amino acids esters as potential chemotherapeutic agents. *Braz J. Med. Biol. Res.* **20**(6), 665.
- Rocha, H. (1982) WHO *Conference Proceed.* Nairobi.
- Rogers, M.R., Popper, S.J. and Worth, D.F. (1990) Amplification of kinetoplast DNA as a tool in the detection and diagnosis of Leishmania. *Exp. Parasitol.* **71**, 267.
- Sacks, D.L., Kenney, R.T., Kreutzer, R.D., Jaffe, C.L., Gupta, A.K., Sharma, M.C., Sinha, S.P., Neva, F.A. and Saran, R. (1995) Indian kala-azar caused by Leishmania tropica. *Lancet* **345**, 959.
- Sarkar, S., Mukherjee, T., Patra, P., Bhaduri, A.N. (1992) Antileishmanial activity of hamycin: a polyene antibiotic. *Biochem. Biophys. Res. Commun.* **182**, 86.

Chapter - 13

Role of Environmental Factors in Etiology of Viral Infection and their Control Measures

*Triveni Krishnan**

Abstract

A thought to ponder........the Ganga has been rated as one of the most polluted rivers in the world. A World Commission on water report states that only three percent of the Ganga water is safe to drink. The water levels in the river are so depleted and polluted that the Sunderbans wetlands and the mangrove forests in the Gangetic delta face a serious threat of extinction. The study supported by the World Bank and the United Nations, discovered that more than half the world's rivers are severely polluted or are rapidly drying up. Commissioned to find ways of ensuring the world's water supply in the 21st century, the research revealed that last year, for the first time, the number of refugees created by environmental factors far exceeded the number of those displaced by war- "the land and water crisis in river basins contributed to the total of 25 million environmental refugees" the report states, adding: "by 2025, the number of environmental refugees could quadruple." Along with the Ganga, the Yellow river in China, the Colorado in the US, the Volga in Russia and the Nile in Africa were found to be the most polluted. Agricultural and industrial waste are the major causes of the pollution. Among the cleanest and healthiest rivers, according to the report, are the Amazon in Brazil and the river Congo in Africa.

[reported to the Asian Age 1, December 1999 by a London correspondent]

Introduction

With the modern advances introduced into the life style, infections are more likely than ever before, to reach vast numbers of people within a very short time. Over the years human beings have begun to move rapidly from place to place, and as the

* Division of Virology, National Institute of Chlolera and Enteric Diseases, Beliaghata, Kolkata-700 010.

transportation of animals and other products for various reasons is becoming quite regular, diseases have been seen to occur in course of new explorations, trade, or warfare. Along with the movement of people, animals, or goods mankind has inadvertently brought far flung species from geographically isolated regions to introduce new microbes into new boundaries. The spread of bubonic plague by rats into Europe from Central Asia and mosquitoes carrying yellow fever from West Africa to the New World afford some examples of disease transmission in bygone days. The availability of trucks and jet aeroplanes have now largely improved the speed of travel between different places and provide much richer opportunities for introducing new infections as seen through global pandemics of certain infections within a short period of their first report. The steady increase of the density of city populations owing to migration of workers into cities from rural areas has shown that diseases spread rapidly through close contact in numerous day care centres, made for the growing children of employed parents.

Infectious diseases are a major problem in developing as well as developed countries and improved diagnosis treatment as well as implementation of suitable preventive and control measures to check their spread is the ultimate goal of researchers world-wide. (Monath and Nasidi, 1993) There has been immense advancement in the areas of detection of viral etiological agents and their molecular characterization during the past few decades with the wide - spread use of PCR [Polymerase Chain Reaction] and sequencing of genomes from newly emerging viruses. Long believed to be all but conquered, infectious diseases have returned with a vengeance. Their return is being felt not only by deadly outbreaks of Ebola in Africa and the worldwide AIDS epidemic but also as Lyme disease, cholera, new strains of influenza, and hantavirus pulmonary syndrome which causes death from respiratory failure, in over half the people infected.

Improved and rapid laboratory diagnosis is very crucial and here researchers have helped by developing efficient new methods, although the resources to make effective use of those methods are often lacking in developing countries. Although diagnosing viral infections can be tedious and tricky, nowadays in many laboratories facilities exist for detection of viruses once the virus has been identified. The ELISA, or "enzyme-linked immunosorbent assay" technique can be performed by trained personnel as routine screening with some caution of eliminating false positives using commercially available kits, or those kits which are distributed free of cost through national surveillance programmes. In these tests, clinical material such as blood from a person who might be infected is typically exposed to components of a virus or other infecting agent to check if their body has reacted by producing proteins called antibodies to combat a specific agent [viral or other agent]. If the body has indeed manufactured the proteins, the person is found to test positive and deemed to have been infected.

The polymerase chain reaction technology (PCR), which allows large quantities of DNA to be synthesized from a single molecule, using appropriate primers and a thermal cycler detects viruses with exquisite sensitivity, speed and specificity. Not only are tests like ELISA and PCR rapid and reliable; they have been made widely available as well, since the essential reagents can frequently be obtained commercially and stored under suitable conditions.

Viral gastroenteritis is rated as one of the most serious problems and is commonly associated with diarrhoea and or vomiting among children and adults during the winter months and also during the monsoon period. These viral infections are a major cause of morbidity among infants in developed countries. On the other hand, in developing countries it is a greater problem causing morbidity as well as mortality in the paediatric age group (*Bhattacharya et al.* 1995). The situation is quite grim during an outbreak and mostly is a result of the over population encountered in most of these settings. Some of the important things to cope up with under demanding situations are as follows : management of dehydration through oral rehydration therapy or intravenous fluid administration, trying to arrange for ready availability of medicines for treatment of the sick and make substitutions for lack of adequate patient care facilities.

A few of the agents recognized as diarrhoeagenic viruses are given below :

(A) Rotaviruses (Das *et al.* 2002; Kapikian *et al.* 2001; Kobayashi *et al.* 2001; Krishan *et al.*1989; 1994, 1996, 1997, 1999; Rupprecht C.E. *et al.* 1995; Vaughn and Hoke, 1995).
(B) Calicivirus (Norwalk-like virus, Sapporo-like-virus), (Green K.Y., 2001)
(C) Astrovirus (Matsui and Greenberg, 2001)
(D) Small Round Viruses (Krishnan T, 1989)
(E) Adenovirus [type 40, 41] (Horwitz M.S., 2001)
(F) Breda virus (Horzinek and Toroviruses, 1993; Krishnan and Naik, 1997)

For viruses potentially transmitted by water, a warm environment attended by poor sanitation and faecal contamination clearly enhances the degree of exposure and the efficiency of transmission. Viruses excreted via the gastrointestinal tract usually infects other susceptible persons via the oral-intestinal route through faecally contaminated hands, food, water, milk, flies, thermometers or other means. Viruses spread via these routes are subject to a greater level of environmental control. In tropical areas and during the summer season in temperate regions, a glorious opportunity for transmission of gastrointestinal infection prevails through frequent contact with water eg. during swimming and drinking from the polluted areas. Infections by Rhinoviruses are also often traced back to seafood or water. Hepatitis A viruses and Hepatitis E viruses are stable viruses in water and if present in sufficient dosage, cannot be inactivated by ordinary levels of chlorine. Moreover, Hepatitis A virus or Human Caliciviruses can persist in oysters and clams over long periods. This poses a very special hazard as such delicacies are often eaten without having been cooked. Adoption of good personal hygiene, especially washing of hands after defecation, proper cleanliness and cooking of food, pasterurization of milk, good waste disposal and purification of drinking water supplies are effective preventive measures.

Other important enteric viruses are Poliomyelitis, ECHO, Coxsackie, Hepatitis A & E and these viruses rarely produce evidence of local disase as a consequence of their multiplication in cells lining the area. Thus diarrhoea, vomiting and abdominal pain are highly unusual features of infection with these agents. Instead, their major target organs and the site of major symptomatology are at a fair distance apart; viz. hepatitis viruses in the liver and enteroviruses in the central nervous system and skin.

D.A. Henderson, who spearheaded the successful smallpox eradication program at WHO, recommended "look out" centers in the expanding urban areas on the periphery of tropical cities. Important port cities and other major places of high population density and flux should also be targeted. Another sensible action would be to include health surveillance in the plans for major projects such as irrigation, road building, and land clearance, especially in areas of high biodiversity. In the longer run, broader surveillance of ecological changes that might presage an increase in natural hosts for disease could also be considered. Epidemics of viral infections result from person to person spread, particularly through the respiratory route in open communities, and in health or extended care facilities. Another crucial point ie. effect of climate on common viral diseases is exerted on the social behaviour of the host. Warm weather also brings closer contact with insect vectors of arboviruses and with dogs and other animal sources of rabies. In the relatively cooler seasons, people mingle indoors thereby promoting transmission of airborne and droplet borne infections. The prevailing environment within most houses and buildings tends to be warm and dry which impairs protective mechanisms of human mucosal surfaces and may permit easier entry and attachment of certain respiratory viruses.

Vector borne spread also accounts for a significant portion of epidemic viral infections all over the world. For infections that require an insect vector, the environment exerts an obvious role in restriction of occurrence of infection and disease to such areas which afford proper temperature, humidity, vegetation, amplifying animal hosts etc. to allow the insect derive a protective habitat. Mosquitoes, flies, ticks and other insects might transmit viral infections in two ways - [a] either passively or [b] through involvement of stages of replication of the virus. During the passive transmission the role of the insect involves simply enabling the virus to be retained on the insect after picking it up from skin leisions or blood viz poliomyelitis or hepatitis. The second type involves arthropod-borne infections such as yellow fever [*Aedes aegypti*] mosquitoes, equine encephalitis etc.] that have in common, replication in both arthropods and vertebrate hosts and transmission between vertebrate animals by the bites of mosquitoes, ticks, sandflies and midges. Some of the dreaded infections, like Acquired Immunodeficiency Disease Syndrome [AIDS], have been derived from viruses that have simply moved into new areas or acquired new hosts. Many are zoonotic, meaning that they have come from animal sources, and they often emerge as the resultant trait of unfavourable ecological changes. Frequently human activities are at the root of such changes-clearing of forests, feeding pastures or cultivating land, for example, can disturb the habitats of natural hosts in these regions such as mice and mosquitoes or other animals, increasing their contact with humans. These infections are closely monitored by the network of World Health Organization [WHO] Arboviruses and Haemorrhagic Fevers Collaborating Centers, which have specialized in unusual infections. Arboviruses which are transmitted by mosquitoes and other arthropods are responsible for diseases such as yellow fever and dengue, and haemorrhagic fevers are those like Ebola that involve massive bleeding. The Ebola virus and quite possibly HIV originated in Africa, one of the most biologically diverse places on Earth and has gradually spread out into other human populations in different parts of the world.

Role of the murine reservoir is seen in the recent emergence of hantavirus from USA and emphasizes the transmission potential of continuous indirect and incidental contact with animals carrying human pathogens. In May 1993 an inexplicable disease was found among hospitalized patients in three different states of USA viz. New Mexico, Arizona and Colorado who were suffering from fever and acute respiratory distress and it ultimately claimed the lives of several patients. Soon the public health system began to co-ordinate every angle and necessary steps required were taken to get as much information that could be acquired from clinicians and the laboratory investigations. This serious pursuit together with the state health department, doctors and people afforded an example that an unknown infectious disease could be tackled with speed and efficiency through the co-operation of various people. The preliminary laboratory tests revealed that the viral infection was of rodent origin and immediately local rodents were captured for further investigation. The host was subsequently identified as a "common deer mouse" which had spread the dangerous viral infection among humans which was called the "hantavirus pulmonary syndrome". The wandering rodents were thereafter controlled and people in the community were educated to protect themselves from such rodents. This Hantavirus outbreak is a classical example of how the external environment exerts its influence on the agent itself, the manner of spread and on the nature of the host response to infection.

There is growing evidence that viral infections, including retroviruses, may be implicated in human diabetes and researchers are looking for more evidence of the association between viruses, such as rubella and Coxsackie B4, with the development of diabetes. The incidence of emerging zoonotic infections has also grown with viruses from animals infecting humans or vice versa. New strategies are necessary for studying diabetogenic agents viz. the viruses, and the future development of programs directed to study interactions between these and the immune system will definitely bring forth very useful information. Under some circumstances autoimmunity could be induced, modulated, or triggered by viruses, and researchers are seeking useful animal models for further investigation. Much more is to be researched upon to understand the roles played by both acute or chronic viral infections and the overall influence of diet and toxins in the patients with diabetes. The association between congenital rubella and incidence of diabetes indicates that Type 1 diabetes is 100 fold greater in these infected cases than the general population. Further studies are necessary to bring about significant correlation as neither vaccine induced infection or natural disease are associated with diabetes. Although rubella provides strong evidence of viral etiology of diabetes, scientists are yet to determine the mode of destruction of beta cells in the system by the virus.

Hepatitis A virus (HAV) poses a serious health problem in developing as well as developed countries. The virus causes infection in the paediatric age group as well as adults and sometimes infects more than 80% of the population in many developing countries by late adolescence. The disease manifests itself as asymptomatic infection in under five year old children but as an acute and self limiting infection among older children and adults. Since 1994, the commercially available cell culture derived inactivated viral vaccine against Hepatitis A is widely used and easily affords protection to the vaccinees against infection. (Innis B. L *et al.* 1994; Werzberger A *et-al.* 1992) Children over two years and those who were routinely vaccinated were protected and the level of infection has dramatically reduced showing that sustained vaccination could possibly eliminate the chances of infection. (Morbidity and Mortality Weekly Report, 1993; Hadler S. C., 1991). Although the vaccine is cost effective it is beneficial for use among high risk populations living in areas which are prone to high levels of infection. The vaccine has also been successful when given to the population at the point of epidemics and during outbreaks for checking the transmission of the virus. It is recognised that the Hepatitis A vaccine is expensive to be distributed to the people of developing countries. Moreover the Hepatitis A vaccine is yet to be included in the Expanded Programme For Immunization [EPI] as there is no suitable vaccine formulation still available for use in infancy or early childhood. Further research into this area is highly essential to develop suitable model for Hepatitis A vaccination in developing countries and preparation of formulations that may be administered to the infant group below two years. It is seen that the efficacious vaccine is quite safe and may also be used with other vaccines for immunization programmes in older age groups. It is important to track down geographical regions and attempt elimination of Hepatitis A infections from such places using suitable strategies to control unwanted infection. It is also highly essential to develop facilities for evaluation of Hepatitis A versus Hepatitis B infection by distinguishing viral hepatitis cases into Hepatitis A or B. With coordinated efforts it will soon be possible to eradicate Hepatitis A infection and studies should be initiated in this direction among widely scattered places to eliminate chances of Hepatitis A among the different populations (Lemon S. M., 1945; Shapiro and Margolis, 1994).

Hepatitis B Virus poses a very serious problem affecting millions of people worldwide and usually tends to be a chronic infection acquired during early part of the life which continues into the adult phase manifesting as liver cancer and ultimately causes death among many of the infected adults in developing countries. Hepatitis B has been reported from several developing as well as developed countries viz. African countries, The Pacific Islands, parts of South America, Asia, New Zealand, Australia USA and poses tremendous threat as the economic burden is felt worldwide through loss of adult lives. Hepatitis B infection can be prevented through immunization prior to or post exposure to the virus. Immunization programmes in wide spread geographical regions afford marked reduction in transmission of new infections, drastic reduction in the number of chronic carriers among routinely immunised cohorts of populations including all age groups from infancy to adulthood. The Hepatitis B vaccine can be administered with other vaccines at the same time and has been successfully included in the Expanded Programme For Immunization [EPI] (Maynard *et al.* 1989). If the first dose of Hepatitis B vaccine could be administered at birth a gradual eradication of Hepatitis B infection may be witnessed at the global level. The widespread distribution of Hepatitis B vaccine for setting up of immunization programs among infants through the generous support of non governmental organizations, health support foundations and funding agencies might expedite the eradication of the Hepatitis B virus thereby reducing the level of hepatocellular carcinoma deaths among adults in future. The costly vaccine may prove to be dear for mass scale immunization in developing countries and it is also necessary to vaccinate the members of families for protection to be maintained in any serious attempt to eradicate the virus. The early monitoring for Hepatitis B infection is an essential step to reduce the spread of infection through ignorant use of infected blood for transfusions etc. and commercially available detection kits can be used to detect infected individuals to evaluate the carrier status and thereby prevent spread of infection. The overall education in guarding against Hepatitis B infection and availability of Hepatitis B vaccine for immunization at the early phase of an individual's life may reduce the chances of infection to the minimum level and these practices should continue into successive generations until the virus is eradicated in the future. It is therefore highly desired that the close monitoring for prompt detection of etiology of any viral hepatitis and particularly Hepatitis B infection should be enforced through surveillance programmes. Further, improved vaccines which may require fewer doses to afford protection may be developed in future. If a suitable vaccine can be developed for oral administration, it would prove very useful and tests to detect variants of Hepatitis B that could be resistant to vaccine induced antibody are future goals to address so as to bring an end to Hepatitis B infection at large, in a global scale.

Measles virus is easily transmitted and highly contagious and is recognized as the eighth leading cause of death among children aged below five years worldwide. The infection can be prevented by a single dose of vaccine given to a child at the age of 9 months [protection efficiency equivalent to 85% for single dose of vaccine or even upto 95% for two doses]. The successful immunization practice coupled with the fact that humans are the only known reservoir, every effort is being taken to successfully eradicate the measles virus in the near future (Oliv J. M., 1994). The two geographical locales interested in the early eradication are the Americas and Eastern Mediterranean while the European region, China and other South African and Pacific Islands have set their goals towards eradication in the near future. Owing to its highly contagious nature, such eradication programs will have to be achieved in a very short time frame through global coordination of efforts to reach time-bound target dates, for its successful eradication. As the Poliomyelitis eradication program was successful through various concerted efforts, the measles virus eradication in developed countries may be achieved by all round strategic support from various resources until the target goals are achieved. In developing countries the eradication of measles may be hindered by the poor infrastructure for safeguarding health and cautious surveillance will therefore play a useful role in controlling unwanted transmission. Adequate care should also be provided for safe injections to be given as well as immunization campaigns to be conducted with good results towards elimination of unwanted infections by the virus. The introduction of good surveillance programs in different phases will lead to proper control of transmission and together with immunization programs organised as mass campaigns, among all newborns and other campaigns at periodic intervals to follow the trend of susceptible individuals will eventually check the unwanted spread of infection. The areas to be developed further are to understand the upcoming changes in mode of transmission as the level of immunized individuals climbs up within the community. The trends should be studied among adults and new methods should be designed to monitor susceptibility for the other younger age groups. These observations will be highly essential to mould advanced strategies towards fruitful halt in transmission of the virus. Other important needs include availability of safe administration practices during immunization, new alternate modes of delivering vaccine at a young age and a reliable assay to evaluate field samples at site for early diagnosis to monitor prevalence.

Rubella virus is chiefly known for causing congenital rubella syndrome in newborns in both developed as well as developing countries. The effect can be observed as impaired hearing, cardiac defects, inflammatory lesions of different organs, cataract formation, and also mental retardation in children born to mothers who were infected during early months of their pregnancy. It is also known to be a major cause of miscarriages and still births among infected pregnant women in their first trimester. Humans are the only known reservoir for rubella and it causes mild to asymptomatic infection in adults and children. The safe precaution is to be immunized with the effective vaccine for rubella and this can be taken along with the measles vaccine. Although the vaccine is effective, rubella is fairly endemic all over the world and the disease burden is realized very strongly in developing countries where susceptible female members of the community have not been properly immunized or have been exposed to wild strains of rubella at some point of time. The initial introduction of data collection on rubella virus can be combined with stringent surveillance programmes in an effort towards implementation of elimination or eradication programs. Thereafter the coverage could yield valuable information to enable reduce infections among high risk populations all over the world. Other important areas of research are to find susceptible groups among adults to check if the age of transmission is shifting. The need for development of suitable laboratory test which could be used in field sites is highly desirable to evaluate the prevalence of infections at large, during epidemiological investigations. For effective eradication of rubella, vaccination programs may be jointly organised so that vaccinees can take the rubella vaccine together with measles vaccine, especially in developing countries. It will be further beneficial to introduce rubella vaccination for pregnant women and other women of child bearing age so as to check congenital rubella syndrome in their newborns. (Cutts F.T. *et al.* 1997; Robertson S. E *et al.* 1997)

Yellow fever virus is spread through mosquitoes and infection can be prevented through administration of the vaccine. (Monath T. P. 1991). The disease is very common in Africa, South America and poses a serious threat of spreading into other neighbouring countries (Monath T. P., 1997). The implementation of vaccination programs in endemic areas and administration of the vaccine to humans visiting countries wherein infection is possible can reduce the level of infection. Such a gradual expansion of immunization programs and sustained surveillance for early detection of infection can be very useful to demarcate location of viral prevalence around the world. The vaccine is protective against different strains of the virus and also found to be safe and is quite effective following a single dose of the vaccine. The vaccine can also be produced in a country where there is a risk of infection with proper guidelines for manufacture and quality control according to international standards. The global immunization program is still lacking for yellow fever due to limited distribution of the strains in defined regions in different parts of the world (Monath and Nasidi, 1993). South America poses a risk of urban epidemics in areas where the *Aedes aegypti* mosquitoes are found which is the principal transmission agent of the virus. The disease could also be transmitted into Asia and countries in the Pacific region through rapid movement of the agents of transmision or through infected people visiting other countries from South America or Africa leading to new epicdemics in these countries. The immediate steps required for efficient control of the spread of yellow fever is to ensure that travellers are properly vaccinated, the children in African countries are immunized, the populations in South America where sylvatic yellow fever exists can be properly immunized and the prevalence of disease can be eventually reduced until it is eliminated from regions of usual prevalence. As yellow fever is found in animal reservoirs the eradication of yellow fever will not be feasible at present. (Pan American Health Organization, 1986; Robertson S E). *et al.* 1996)

Rabies virus is spread through bites and saliva of animals such as dogs in urban areas in different parts of the world and also red foxes found in parts of Eastern Canada or Western Europe (Rupprecht *et al.*, 1995; Smith, 1995). As the animal reservoir is chiefly involved, the disease cannot be eradicated easily and control of the spread of rabies infection in these animal reservoirs will eventually be able to reduce mortality and morbidity for humans. (Hanlon and Rupprecht, 1998; Meslin F-X, 1994). An essential component of effective rabies post-exposure prophylaxis includes rabies immuno globulin, which is frequently in short supply and too costly for routine use in many developing countries. As post exposure prophylaxis is expensive, therefore reduction of rabies infections among animal reservoirs have to be tackled with proper planning as different animals and their habitats have to be studied for prevalence and strategic planning is essential for fruitful rabies control (Morbidity and Mortality Weekly Report, 1991). A good example of rabies control in wild animals eg. red foxes in Eastern Canada and Western Europe was achieved through the use of oral baited vaccines. (Baer G.M., 1988; Morbidity and Mortality Weekly Report, 1997) Such a program should be coordinated from the health department, agriculture department and the environment protection agencies to move actively and set up immunization programs to protect human and animals for reducing the level of exposure towards rabies infection. Licensed cell-culture-based vaccines are available for veterinary and human use and also prevalence of infection can be monitored through testing for antigenic and genomic markers associated with animal host reservoirs. Humans facing higher risk for rabies, such as veterinarians, other persons with vocational risk, and members of certain occupational groups, should be immunized prior to exposure. The utmost priority for research into rabies should be enforced to include development of a safe and effective vaccine for mass immunization of dogs and other animal reservoirs, such as an oral bait vaccine,which will be treatable in case of any inadvertent ingestion by children. Replacement of brain-derived vaccines, which cause neurological reactions should be done with existing cell-culture based vaccines. It is of vital importance to ensure the safety and efficacy of currently manufactured rabies vaccines, since, in some instances, production and quality control is unsatisfactory for many of the indigenous rabies vaccine from developing countries and the vaccine is not upto prescribed international standards. There should be a serious drive to identify economical, effective alternatives to human rabies immunoglobulin. There should be an overall development for the better understanding of all aspects of rabies transmission in bats, which has now emerged as the most important cause of rabies in the USA and is the only recognized native rabies reservoir in Australia. Recent discoveries of previously unknown bat reservoirs of rabies virus underscore the importance of continued research to define the natural history of the disease. (Allworth *et al.* 1996). Concurrently, existing knowledge of the virology of rhabdoviruses should be applied to develop safe and effective antiviral compounds that could be integrated into existing post-exposure regimens of passive and active immunization. Moreover, advancing control measures to safeguard wildlife against rabies through oral vaccination, continued development of novel vaccines, baits, and baiting strategies is required to combat rabies in future.

Japanese encephalitis is transmitted from natural reservoirs and can only be controlled or eliminated by administering suitable vaccines to the population at risk of exposure to infection (Rojanosuphot and Tsai, 1995). In Asia the disease is a major cause of permanent neurological sequelae among infected children and thereby poses yet another serious public health problem. The infections have gradually been spreading into many different parts of Asia and have also been reported from other countries in Australia and Pacific regions. (Mackenzie J. S *et al.* 1997; Vaughn and Hoke, 1992) The use of vaccine for protection through childhood immunization programs has enabled the disease to be nearly eliminated from Japan, Taiwan and Republic of Korea. There has been remarkable reduction in annual incidence of infection in Thailand also ever since the Japanese encephalitis vaccine was introduced into the Expanded Program For Immunization [EPI]. (Burke and Leake, 1988; Morbidity and Mortality Weekly Report, 1993). In addition to infant vaccination programs, interruption of viral transmission in the animal reservoir can be reduced by vaccinating or removing pigs or by vector control as an adjunct strategy to check spread of viral infection. The current effective vaccine is derived from infected mouse brain and requires two doses for primary immunization and numerous booster doses to maintain immunity. The vaccine is also reported to cause hypersensitivity reactions in 0.5% of vaccinees. (Plesner and Ronne,

1997) The fact that vaccine production, supply, and cost is limited by the technical complexity of the manufacturing process is of serious concern and efforts are still on to provide a satisfactory method of controlling the viral infection. For many developing countries, lack of resources limits the use of vaccine despite political will to implement the vaccine into national programmes. An alternative, live attenuated vaccine, produced and distributed in China, is safe and effective and has been used in more than 100 million children. (Hennessy S. *et al.* 1996) Despite requiring two doses, the vaccine could be available at a lower cost than the current vaccine; however, it is currently licensed only in China.

The appropriate definition for eradication and elimination of infectious diseases was adopted during the Dahlem Workshop on the Eradication Of Infectious Diseases. When incidence of any disease has reduced to zero level within a defined geographical area with continued application of intervention measures as required, the control of disease at such a stage is called "elimination" and only permanent world wide reduction of any disease to zero level without any intervention measures is referred to as "eradication". Over the years several viruses such as measles, rubella and Hepatitis B have emerged as primary candidates to concentrate upon for their early eradication. Neither the Hepatitis A virus can be eradicated or eliminated at the present, nor other viruses which harbour in animal reservoirs such as rabies virus, yellow fever virus or Japanese encephalitis virus can be eradicated. However adequate measures can be applied to control the spread of these viruses primarily in the environment or through properly planned immunization programmes so as to achieve elimination of such viral infections among human populations. A wide range of viral infections are encountered owing to their diverse epidemiological features and different mechanisms of viral pathogenesis. Hence a common, suitable approach for control of all viral infections is lacking and each virus is to be addressed according to its special properties for effective control or management. Important milestones achieved till date in virus research have seen the spectacular development of suitable vaccines for controlling some of the viral infections; moreover the eradication of vectors after their detection and improved sanitation practices have also led to significant control in spread of viral infection in the community for some viruses. The development of antivirals for treatment of some viral infections is a great achievement. Tireless efforts are continuously directed to alleviate suffering through successful development of new methodologies for effective control of viral infections.

Since the public health infrastructure in many countries of the world is still lacking or rather rudimentary, it is still unable to absorb large investments for a modest beginning, the initial costs of implementing the international components of an early warning and response system for infectious diseases could be modest with investment of few millions per year. Such funds could be made available from pooling together the resources of different countries; the rest could be collected from private donations and other leading organizations that have generously contributed to public health programs in the past such as the World Bank, other development agencies, and major foundations interested in such upcoming efforts for safeguarding mankind from infliction by diseases. The money would finance upgraded resources at a few chosen locations, supplying office support and items such as computers with appropriate software for collection and disssemination of useful information. The setting up of modern communication facilities such as telephone or satellite links will ensure reliable data gathering and communications into a chosen terminal. The infrastructure would be ably run by some personnel with adequate training, reporting to consortium members, and a small central staff as well who could report on the achievement and plan for further improvement.

The allocation of budget for protecting the environment and safeguarding public health as a priority is to be well planned and funds are to be managed cautiously to achieve useful goals. The infrastructure to monitor disease and good patient care in hospitals and networking of the country's surveillance programmes are available in few developed countries and are still only in their infancy in other developing countries. The first step to initiate such useful monitoring should address the early detection of emerging and re-emerging infectious diseases in the respective zone and thereafter arrange for quick dissemination of useful information across network of clinicians and health care personnel.

As we ponder and assess the present situation it is clear that human beings are vulnerable to innumerable viral or other infections. As we are only in the process of establishing surveillance programmes to detect emerging infections at an early stage in small pockets across the world, the urgent need for a global surveillance system is felt deeply. The timely response to the early detection will be an added boon when we realize the staggering costs of management of diseases after they have established themselves in host populations. Hence all concentrated efforts should be directed to develop adequate surveillance and response programmes according to the facilities available in different regions or geographical locales and the rewards will be felt if mankind is exposed to fewer diseases in the future with increased knowledge to safeguard his environment and weed out the factors which cause harm or infection.

References

- Allworth A, Murray K, Morgan J. (1996). A human case of encephalitis due to a lyssavirus recently identified in fruit bats. *Communicable diseases intelligence* **20** : 504.
- Baer G. M. (1988). Oral rabies vaccination : an overview. *Reviews of Infectious Diseases,* **10** (Suppl. 4) : S644-S648.
- Bhattacharya S. K., M. K. Bhattacharya, B. Manna, D. Dutta, A. Deb, P. Dutta, A. G. Goswami, A. Dutta, S. Sarkar, A. Mukhopadhaya, Triveni Krishnan, T. N. Naik and G. B. Nair (1995). Risk factors for development of dehydration in young children with acute watery diarrhoea. *Acta Paediatrica* **84** : 160-164 (Scandinavia).
- Burke D. S, Leake C. J.(1988). Japanese encephalitis. In : Monath TP. ed. The arboviruses : *Epidemiology and Ecology,* Vol. III. Boca Raton, CRC Press, 63-92.
- Morbidity and Mortality Weekly Report, Centers for Disease Control and Prevention. Rabies Prevention -- United States, (1991): *Recommendations of the Immunization Practices Advisory Committee* (ACIP). 40 (RR-3) : 1-19.
- Morbidity and Mortality Weekly Report, Centers for Disease Control and Prevention. Inactivated Japanese encephalitis virus vaccine. *Recommendations of the Advisory Committee on Immunization Practices* (ACIP) (1993), 42 (RR-1).
- Morbidity and Mortality Weekly Report, Centers for Disease Control and Prevention. Prevention of Hepatitis A through active or passive immunization. *Recommendations of the Advisory Committee on Immunization Practices.* (1996), 45 (RR-15) : 1-30.
- Morbidity and Mortality Weekly Report, Centers for Disease Control and Prevention. Compendium of animal rabies control, 1997. National Association of State Public Health Veterinarians, Inc. *Morbidity and Mortality* Weekly Report, (1997), 46 : 1-9.
- Cutts F. T. *et al.* (1997). Control of rubella and congenital rubella syndrome (CRS) in developing countries. 1: Burden of disease from CRS. *Bulletin of the World Health Organization,* **75** : 55-68.

- Das S, A Sen, G. Uma, V. Varghese, S. Chauduri, S. K. Bhattacharya, T. Krishan, P. Dutta, D. Dutta, M. K. Bhattacharya, U. Mitra N. Kobayashi, T. N. Naik (2002). Gemonic diversity of Group A rotavirus strains infecting humans in Eastern India. *Journal of Clinical Microbiology* **40** [1]: 146-149, [ASM,USA]
- Green K. Y., Chanock R. M. and Kapikian A. Z. (2001). *Human Caliciviruses In Fields Virology* Chief Eds D. M. Knipe and P. M. Howley, Lippincott Williams and Wilkins , USA : Vol I, Chapter 27, pp. 841-874.
- Hadler S. C. (1991). *Global impact of Hepatitis* A virus infection changing patterns. In : Hollinger. FB *et al.* eds. Viral hepatitis and liver disease. Baltimore, MD, Williams & Wilkins, : 14-20.
- Hanlon C. A, Rupprecht C. E. (1998). The reemergence of rabies. In : Scheld W. M *et al.* eds. *Emerging infections*, Washington, DC, ASM Press : 59-80.
- Hennessy S. *et al.* (1996). Effectiveness of live-attenuated Japanese encephalitis vaccine (SA14-14-2) : a case-control study. *Lancet* **347** :1583-1586.
- Horwitz M. S. (2001). *Adenoviruses. In Fields Virology* Chief Eds D. M. Knipe and P. M. Howley, Lippincott Williams and Wilkins, USA : Vol. II, Chapter 68, pp. 2301-2326.
- Horzinek M. C.(1993). Toroviruses. In Webster R. G., Granoff A. editors. *Encyclopedia of Virology* Vol. III London : Academic Press. 1452-1458.
- Innis B. L *et al.* (1994). Protection against Hepatitis A by an inactivated vaccine. *Journal of the American Medical Association,* **271** : 1328-1334.
- Kapikian A. Z., Hoshino Y. and Chanock R. M. (2001). *Rotaviruses In Fields Virology* Chief Eds D. M. Knipe and P. M. Howley, Lippincott Williams and Wilkins, USA : Vol. II, Chapter 55, pp. 1787-1833.
- Kobayashi, T. N. Naik, Y. Kusuhara, T. Krishnan, A. Sen, S. K. Bhattacharya, K. Taniguchi, M. M. Alam, T. Urasawa and S. Urasawa (2001). Sequence analysis of genes encoding structural and nonstructural proteins of a human group B rotavirus detected in Calcutta, India. *"J. Medical Virology"* **64** (4) : 583-588, 2001 [Wiley-Liss, Inc.]
- Krishnan T, T. N. Naik, A. Curry, S. K. Bhattacharya, P. Dutta, D. Dutta and S. C. Pal (1989). Electron microscopic detection of diarrhoeagenic viruses from infants and children in Eastern India. Proceedings of the Indo-UK Workshop on Diarrhoeal Diseases, National Institute of Cholera & Enteric Diseases, *Indian Council of Medical Research,* pp. 12-21 (India).
- Krishnan, T., B. Burke, S. Shen, T. N. Naik and U. Desselberger (1994). Molecular epidemiology of human rotaviruses in Manipur

: genome analysis of rotaviruses of long electropherotype and subgroup I. *Archives of Virology* **134** : 279-292, (Springer Verlag, Austria).

- Krishnan T, T. N. Naik and U. Desselberger (1996). Molecular epidemiology of human rotaviruses : reassortment in vivo as mechanism for strain diversity ? *Journal of Infection* **32** : 169-170, (UK).
- Krishnan T. & T. N. Naik (1997). Electronmicroscopic evidence of torovirus like particles in children with diarrhoea. *Indian J. Med. Res.* **105** : 108-110.
- Krishnan T, A. Sen, J. Sinha Choudhury, S. Das, T. N. Naik, S. K. Bhattacharya (1999). Emergence of adult diarrhoea rotavirus in Calcutta, India. *The Lancent* **353** : 380-381 of 30, January [UK].
- Lemon S. M. (1985). Type A viral hepatitis : new developments in an old disease. *New England Journal of Medicine,* **313** : 1059-1067.
- Mackenzie J. S *et al.* (1997). Emergence of Japanese encephalitis virus in the Australasian region. In : Salluzzo J. F, Dodet B. eds. *Factors in the emergence of arbovirus diseases.* Paris, Elsevier, 191-201.
- Matsui S. M. and Greenberg H. B. (2001). *Astroviruses.* In Fields Virology Chief Eds D. M. Knipe and P. M. Howley, Lippincott Williams and Wilkins, USA Vol. I, Chapter 28, pp. 875-893.
- Maynard J. E., Kane M. A., Hadler S. C. (1989). Global control of hepatitis B through vaccination : role of Hepatitis B vaccine in the Expanded Programme on Immunization. *Reviews of Infectious Diseases,* 11: s 574-578.
- Meslin F-X, Fishbein D. B, Matter H. C. (1994). Rationale and prospects for rabies elimination in developing countries. In : Rupprecht C. E. *et al.* eds. *Current topics in Microbiology and Immunology,* Berlin, Springer-Verlag, 1-26.
- Monath T. P. (1991). Yellow fever : Victor, Victoria? Conqueror, Conquest? Epidemics and research in the last 40 years and prospects for the future. *American Journal of Tropical Medicine and Hygiene,* **45** : 1-43.
- Monath T. P., Nasidi A (1993). Should yellow fever vaccine be included in the Expanded Programme of Immunization in Africa? A cost-effectiveness analysis. *American Journal of Tropical Medicine and Hygiene,* **48** : 274-299.
- Monath T. P. (1997). Epidemiology of yellow fever: current status and speculations on future trends. In : Saluzzo J. F, Dodets G. eds. *Factors in the emergence of arbovirus diseases.* Paris, Elsevier : 143-156.
- Murray C. J. L., Lopez A. D. eds., (1996). The global burden of disease: a comprehensive assessment of mortality and disability from diseases, injuries, and risk factors in 1990 projected to 2020 -- *summary.* Geneva, World Health Organization, 17-26.

- Oliv J. M., Aylward B. R, Melgaard B (1997). Disease eradication as a public health strategy : is measles next? *World Health Statistic Quarterly,* **50** : 185-187.
- Pan American Health Organization (1986). Present status of yellow fever : Memorandum from a PAHO meeting. *Bulletin of hte World Health Organization,* **64** : 511-524.
- Plesner A. M, Ronne T. (1997). Allergic mucocutaneous reactions to Japanese encephalitis vaccine. *Vaccine,* **15** :1239-1243.
- Robertson S. E *et al.*(1996) Yellow fever : a decade of reemergence.*Journal of the American Medical Association,* **276** : 1157-1162.
- Robertson S. E *et al.* (1997). Control of rubella and congenital rubella syndrome (CRS) in developing countries. 2 : Vaccination against rubella. *Bulletin of the World Health Organization,* **75** : 69-80.
- Rojanosuphot S, Tsai T. F. (1995). eds. Regional workshop on control strategies for Japanese encephalitis. *South East Asia Journal of Tropical Medicine and Public Health,* **26** (S3) : 1-59.
- Rupprecht C. E *et al.* (1995). The ascension of wildlife rabies : a cause for public health concern or intervention? *Emerging Infectious Diseases,* **1** : 107-114.
- Sen A. N., Kobayashi, S. Das, Triveni Krishnan, S. K. Bhattacharya, S. Urasawa, T. N. Naik (2000). Amplification of various genes of human Group B rotavirus from stool specimens by RT-PCR. *Journal of Clinical Virology* **17** : 177-181 [Elsevier].
- Sen A. N. Kobayashi, S. Das, Triveni Krishnan, S. K. Bhattachrya, T. N. Naik (2001). The evolution of human Group B rotaviruses. *The Lancet* **357** : 198-199 of 20, January [UK].
- Shapiro C. N, Margolis H. S. (1994). Worldwide epidemiology of hepatitis A virus infection. *Journal of Hepatology,* **18** (suppl. 2) : s 11-14.
- Smith J. S., Orciari L. A, Yager P. A. (1995). Molecular epidemiology of rabies in the United States. *Seminars in Virology,* **6** : 387-400.
- Vaughn D. W, Hoke C. H. (1992). The epidemiology of Japanese encephalitis : prospects for prevention. *Epidemiological Reviews.* **14** : 197-221.
- Werzberger A *et al.* (1992). A controlled trial of formalin-inactivated hepatitis A vaccine in healthy children. *New England Journal of Medicine,* **327** : 453-457.

Section II
Water Borne Diseases

Chapter - 14

Management & Prevention of Acute Diarrhoea

*P Dutta**

Abstract

Acute diarrhoeal diseases are the major cause of morbidity, mortality and hospitalisation among children in the developing countries. According to the nature of diarrhoeal stools, acute diarrhoeas are classified as acute watery (secretory) diarrhoea and acute bloody diarrhoea (dysentery). Vibrio cholerae 01, 0139, enterotoxigenic and enteropathogenic Escherichia coli and rotavirus are the main causative agents of acute watery diarrhoea, while the pathogens producing dysentery include different species of Shigella (S. sonnei, S. flexneri, S. boydii, S. dysenteriae), and Entamoeba histolytica. Rehydration therapy is an essential part of the management of acute watery diarrhoea. Rehydration can be done either orally or by intravenous route according to the degree of dehydration. Home available fluids or oral rehydration salts solution (ORS) should be used at home for prevention of dehydration from the onset of diarrhoea. ORS should be used for correction of initial dehydration and during the maintenance phase in patients who suffer from some dehydration. Ringer's lactate is the ideal intravenous fluid for correction of severe dehydration due to diarrhoea. Antibiotics play a vital role in the management of cholera, shigellosis, amebiasis, giardiasis. Proper feeding during diarrhoea is also recommended.

Introduction

Even today diarrhoeal diseases are a major cause of illness and death among infants and young children, specially in developing countries including India. About half of the childhood mortality is attributed to acute diarrhoeal illness either directly or as a result of

---

* Deputy Director & Head, Division of Clinical Medicine, National Institute of Cholera and Enteric Diseases, Beliaghat, Kolkata-700 010.

various diarrhoea-malnutrition cycles. A nation wide survey by the Registrar General of India in 1978 identified diarrhoea as a major killer and cause of illness among children. It was also estimated that 1.5 million under 5 children die due to diarrhoea each year (Registrar General, 1979). Another survey carried out in 1991 revealed that mortality due to diarrhoea has declined from an estimated 1.5 million in 1978 to about 0.6 to 0.7 million in 1991. (NCSSMP, 1994).

Acute diarrhoea is usually caused by infectious agents. The agents vary according to the nature of diarrhoea e.g. watery (secretory) diarrhoea or dysentery (bloody diarrhoea). Pathogens causing watery diarrhoea include *Vibrio cholerae* (01, 0139 and non-01 non-0139), enterotoxigenic *Escherichia coli,* Rotavirus and others, while the pathogens causing dysentery include various species of Shigella *(S. flexneri, S. sonnei, S. boydii, S. dysenteriae),* Salmonella and *Entamoeba histolytica.* The micro-organisms responsible for such acute diarrhoeal diseases were poorly identified before 1970s. Following recent advances in diagnostic methodology, the causative agents and their pathophysiological mechanism can be identified in most acute diarrhoeal illnesses. Thirty years ago, in many parts of the world including India, the etiology could be accurately assigned in only 20% of all cases. However, by 1999, 35-38 important pathogens causing acute diarrhoea in most of the developing countries including India are identified in nearly 90% of cases (Bhattacharya S K *et al.* 1999). A variety of social, economical, political, technological and environmental factors usually change the pattern of etiological agents of acute diarrhoea from time to time. Like other developing countries etiological agents are also dynamic in India. National surveillance system of enteric pathogens has been set up in most of the developed countries to accumulate the information of infection caused by enteric pathogens nationwide and to identify the priorities for prevention and control of infections. In contrast, our country does not take proper care to develop national surveillance system of enteric pathogens. Recently, there are few crucial observations for understanding of pathophysiology of diarrhoea which facilitate the improved treatment of diarrhoea. Enteric pathogens cause disease either by toxigenic or invasive mechanisms, sometimes both these mechanisms are involved for producing diarrhoea. Organisms such as *Vibrio cholerae* and some *Escherichia coli* multiply in the small intestine producing enterotoxins that cause this organ to secrete fluid and electrolytes but do not cause significant histological damage to the epithelium. The extra fluid produced overwhelm the absorption capacity of the the gastrointestinal tract distal in the site of secretion and more water is therefore passed in the stool which is manifested by diarrhoea (Formal *et al.* 1983). In contrast, invasive pathogens like *Shigellae, Salmonellae,* some *Escherichia coli, Vibrio parahaemolyticus* damage the intestinal mucosa. This mucosal damage, which may range from a mild inflammatory response to gross ulceration, is a consequence of the ability of these pathogens to invade the intestinal epithelium (Formal S B *et al.* 1983) . Some of the invasive organisms may also have characteristics of enterotoxigenic and enteropathogenic organisms. For example, *Shigella dysenteriae* type 1 produces a toxin that is both enterotoxic and cytotoxic and *Salmonella typhimurium* produces a toxin that is antigenically and biologically similar to cholera toxin (choleragen).

Far more important has been the clear cut demonstration that death due to acute diarrhoeal illness, regardless of etiologic agent, can almost always be prevented by adequate correction of intestinal fluid and electrolyte losses, the majority of such illnesses are self-limiting if water and electrolyte depletion is corrected. Also of great importance has been the observation that deprivation of oral nutrition is rather harmful for recovery from acute diarrhoeal illnesses.

Better understanding of the pathophysiology of cholera and other diarrhoeal diseases led us to find that death due to acute diarrhoeal illness, regardless of etiologic agent, can almost always be prevented by adequate correction of intestinal fluid and electrolyte losses, the majority of such illnesses being self-limited. In the past, intravenous fluid therapy was considered the treatment of choice for correcting fluid losses in acute diarrhoeal illnesses in both adults and children. Without evaluating the proper role of antimicrobial agents in acute diarrhoeal diseases, almost all the patients were treated with antimicrobial agents either singly or in combination. The demonstration that orally administered glucose-electrolyte solutions can be life saving in cholera has provided one of the most dramatic and rapid application of a basic scientific observation to clinical medicine (Sachar D B 1965, Hirschhorn N, *et al.* 1968). The concept of use of oral glucose electrolyte solution emerged from the fact that glucose enhances the absorption of sodium and water across the brush border of intestinal epithelium. Moreover, the gut mucosa shows no structural abnormality in most cases of acute watery/secretory diarrhoea and absorption capacity of the gut remains essentially intact (Anonymus, 1978; Sachar DB 1965, Hirschhorn N, *et al.* 1968). Presently it is well documented that oral glucose electrolyte solution is effective in vast majority of actute diarrhoeal illness in all age groups and in all etiologies of diarrhoea (WHO 1990). Use of oral glucose electrolyte solution has revolutionized the treatment of diarrhoeal diseases.

In 1978, The World Health Organization (WHO) started the Control of Diarrhoeal Diseases (CDD) Program globally, with the key strategy of effective case management mainly with a single formula of oral glucose-electrolyte solution (ORS). Till date, about 129 countries throughout the world have participated in CDD programme. The Government of India also launched CDD Programme in 1978 with WHO/UNICEF assistance with the objective of reducing mortality of children due to diarrhoeal diseases. Since 1992-93 this programme has been incorporated into Child Survival and Safe Motherhood (CSSM) programme (Manchanda V.K., 1996). Very recently this programme has become a part of Reproductive Child Health (RCH) programme. The national programme emphasizes more on use of ORS. This programme has also stimulated production and distribution of the packets of ORS, trained thousands of doctors and health workers to use this ORS. Proper use of ORS has also been promoted through mass media to strengthen the case management of diarrhoea of under five children through mothers at domestic level. This programme has also given proper attention for promotion of continued feeding during diarrhoeal episodes. Ensuring availability of ORS packets at health facilities and in the community is also an important aspect of the programme.

WHO and UNICEF want to implement unified and standard case management of diarrhoeal diseases throughout the world. However, several countries adopted CDD programme to combat their own problem, keeping the basic principals intact. The treatment of acute watery diarrhoea without having signs and symptoms of dehydration (normal skin turgor, eyes and thirst, passage of urine normally and child is quiet) is prevention of dehydration by giving more fluid and usual diet. Treatment should be started at home at the time of the onset of diarrhoea by giving home available fluid (HAF) e.g. salt sugar solution, pop rice water, kanji etc. ORS may be given if available at the time of onset of diarrhoea. This hypothesis of use of home available fluid (HAF) was formulated by the Indian scientists that most of the children with diarrhoea in the community do not have dehydration so there is no need to rehydrate them with ORS. However, HAF can easily be prepared by the mothers with the ingredients available at home and can be used safely and effectively to prevent dehydration. Thus it reduces the requirement of ORS (Deb *et al.* 1985). This hypothesis was tested in the field trial in a pilot study using a 3-tier strategy of implementation of ORS and/or HAF at the community level. The concept of oral rehydration therapy (ORT) including the use of a recommended HAF and / or ORS came into existence, which is now the key strategy not only in the National but also in the Global CDD programme (WHO, 1990) . Breast feeding should be continued throughout the episode of diarrhoea in breastfed children. Apart from being nutritious, mother's milk is the fluid of choice for prevention of dehydration in neonates and young children. For young infants whose safe nutrient is animal milk or formula, milk should be continued without diluting them. Older children and adults should continue normal food (cereal, vegetables, pulses and others) which they are habituated to take before diarrhoea.

Patients with "some" dehydration (having the signs and symptoms of sunken eyes, dry mouth, thirst, loss of skin elasticity or irritable behaviour), ORS recommended by WHO should be administered in two phases e.g. rehydration phase (to correct the existing water and electrolyte deficit) and maintenance phase (to replace ongoing losses of water and electrolytes due to continuing diarrhoea in order to prevent occurrence of dehydration). Majority of the cases of "some" dehydration can successfully be managed by ORS recommended by WHO (1990). Even after recommendation of single standard formula of ORS by WHO, some physicians of industrialized countries have often had difficulty in agreeing on the optimal sodium concentration (90 mmol/litre) for fear of producing hypernatraemia in neonates and infants in non-cholera diarrhoea. To overcome this problem scientists from Costa Rica recommended 2 volumes of ORS followed by 1 volume of plain water (2:1 regimen) (Pizarro D *et al.* 1980). However, in Indian situation it was felt that 2:1 regimen could be confusing to the illiterate mothers. In a subsequent study in our country it was observed that uninterrupted breast feeding along with standard ORS could successfully avoid hypernatraemia (Dutta *et al*, 1984). However the children under 6 months of age and not being breastfed should receive other milk food or 100-200 ml clean water. Another study demonstrates that ORS is an effective means of treating acute dehydrating diarrhoeal illness caused by a variety of etiological agents in severely malnourished children, thus, observations originally made in children of varoius nutritional status in the developing countries have been shown to be equally valid in severely malnourished children (Dutta *et al.* 1991). These findings were also incorporated in the National as well as Global CDD programme. Other studies documented that early oral food intake in addition to ORT had no adverse effect on either duration or severity of diarrhoeal illness in the children. Hence the recommendation is that breast feeding should be continued through out the period of illness. Older children and adults should be given food every 3-6 hours from the beginning or as soon as they are hydrated.

Patients with severe dehydration with or without shock, fatigue, stupor or coma, uncontrollable vomiting (>4 times/hours), high purging rate (>15 ml/stool/kg/hour) should be given intravenous Ringer's lactate solution. Ringer's lactate is the preferred solution for all age groups as it contains adequate concentration of sodium, potassium and lactate which is converted to bicarbonate to correct acidosis WHO(1990). Intravenous fluid should be used only for correction of initial dehydration for 6 hours or 3 hours in case of infacts and older children respectively. Maintenance should always be done with ORS except few cases where the stool volume and purging rates are high, having chances of return of signs and symptoms of severe dehydration where intravenous fluid is again indicated.

Still now misconception among the general population in our country has led to the belief that a wide variety of foods should be withheld or markedly reduced during diarrhoea. Many people also avoid milk for fear that children with diarrohea cannot tolerate it. Many of the doctors and health workers of our country often encourage this practice. However recent concept is that breast feeding should not be interrupted during diarrhoea. When cow's milk is used; full strength milk should be fed throughout the disease and in convalescence. The concept of diluting milk with water should be altogether avoided. It has also been suggested that a wide variety of common local food, many of vegetables origin and some with significant contents of vegetable oil, may be used to feed children with diarrhoea.The amount of oil are particularly important to increase the diet's energy density and to provide adequate amount of dietary energy to anorexia children. National CDD Programme has insisted on advantages of continued feeding during diarrhoea for past two decades, inspite of that, withholding food during diarrhoea and substitution of nutritious foods with dilute preparations of low nutritional value are still common practice in our country. Economic factors are another cause of poor dietary practices during diarrhoea. Many of the foods often recommended by doctors are more expensive than those commonly available in low income household. Special diets, such as commercial soy based formulas and elemental or semi-elemental diets are unaffordable in poorer section of the people of rural areas of our country. Availability and cost must be considered in selecting the recommended food.

The proper role of drugs particularly antimicrobial agents in acute diarrhoeal disease has been the subject of much controversy, however, in past all patients with acute diarrhoea were treated with antimicrobial agents and other antidiarrhoeal drugs since the specific cause was rarely determined. Presently it is well known that antibiotics are required for severe cholera and shigellosis only. The antibiotic of choice for severe cholera is tetracycline WHO(1990). Tetracycline may not be available in syrup form for pediatric use in many countries because of fear of staining of teeth and its accumulation in the growing ends of bones. However, most authorities believe that cholera is the only indication of pediatric use of tetracycline WHO(1990). Norfloxacin and ciprofloxacin are highly effective alternatives WHO(1990). Children with cholera may be treated with furazolidone (Karshner *et al.* 1970) or trimethoprim sulphamethoxazole (TMP-SMX) (Bhattacharya *et al.* 1994). Drugs are used as an adjunct to rehydration therapy. They help by reducing stool volume and stop excretion of vibrios in the stool. However, *Vibrio cholerae* 0139 strains isolated in 1992 and recent strains of *Vibrio cholerae* 01 isolated in certain cholera endemics areas are resistant to TMP-SMX and furazolidone (Bhattacharya *et al*, 1993; Mukherjee *et al.* 1996). Erythromycin may be used when recommended antibiotics are not available or resistant to them WHO(1990). Single dose of 300 mg doxycycline can be used in adult cholera patients (De *et al.* 1975)

Shigellosis may be treated with oral ampicillin or TMP-SMX or nalidxic acid for 5 days depending upon the drug susceptibility pattern of local *Shigella* isolates (Bhattacharya *et al.* 1987; Salam *et al.* 1988). However, *Shigella* strains in many countries have developed resistance to nalidixic acid (Khan Samidual 1982) . In such situations norfloxacin or ciprofloxacin may be used in adults (Bhattacharya *et al.* 1991; Binnish *et.al.* 1990). Norfloxacin or ciprofloxacin may also be used for pediatric population as recent studies showed that these drugs do not produce cartilage toxicity in children (Bhattacharya *et al.* 1997). Metronidazole is still the drug of choice for the treatment of amoebiasis and giardiasis WHO(1990). Antimicrobial agents are remarkably effective in the treatment of cholera and shigellosis. The medical profession has been given the responsibility of dispensing the agents for the benefit of patients. However, many of these agents are used indiscrepantly as those are available over the counter in our country. Moreover, many of the national as well as multinational pharmaceutical industries are preparing drugs in different combinations for the treatment of diarrhoea which are mostly unsafe and unnecessary. The medical professionals, by their leadership in the field and in close ties with industry, play a critical role in evaluating antimicrobial agents and making recommendations to the professionals concerning their use. The recommendations involve the best agent for each indication, optimal dose and duration, methods to minimize the development of resistance and consideration of reasonable cost. Certain drugs like charcoal, pectin, kaolin, diphenoxylate with atropine, paragariss, loperamides, cardiotomies, antiemetics and steroids have been said to be useful in the management of diarrhoea, although no studies have confirmed their efficancy WHO, 1990; Bhattacharya *et al.* 1994).

Appropriate and timely treatment is highly efficacious in reducing mortality from diarrhoea, but this cannot reduce the incidence of diarrhoea. Prevention of diarrhoea primarily means preventing the susceptible persons (particularly children at risk) from acquiring diarrhoeal diseases. WHO has given priority to the following strategies and intervention for prevention of diarrhoeal diseases : i) promotion of exclusive breast feeding during first 4-6 months of life. Immunological properties of breast milk helps to protect the infants from infection (Jalliffe D B and Jelliffe E F P 1981). The advantages of breast feeding include that it is clean and does not require the use of bottle, teats, water and formula which is easily contaminated with bacteria that can cause diarrhoea WHO (1990) . ii) Improved weaning practice which require selection of nutritious food for the children more than 4-6 months of age and good hygienic practice like hand washing during preparation and serving food WHO (1990). iii) Risk of diarrhoea can be significantly reduced by using safe and clean water. Water should be protected from contamination. Prevention of contamination of stored water at the household level is also important to cut down the transmission of diarrhoeagenic pathogens WHO (1990); Deb *et al.* (1986). iv) Personal and domestic hygiene like proper hand washing with soap and water before preparing food, before feeding children and during ablution reduces the incidence of diarrhoea (Khan and Samidulla, 1982). Clean domestic and kitchen hygiene is also important for reduction of incidence of diarrhoea WHO (1990). v) Access and use of clean, functioning latrine and proper disposal of stools of both animal and human are essential in preventing the spread of enteropathogens causing diarrhoea WHO (1990). vi) Immunization against measles reduces the incidence of measles related diarrhoeal diseases WHO (1990).

Natural calamities are quite common in our country and during post disaster periods, water supply and sanitation has deteriorated at large. During post flood or post cyclone situations, inaccessibility of safe drinking water sources or improper or unhygienically erected (on emergency basis) hand pumps have been found to be associated with diarrhoeal epidemics. Not only good water supply but also improved sanitary or environmental conditions reduce diarrhoeal morbidity. Use of halogen tablets, solution of bleaching powder or hypochlorite solution may be used for disinfecting water in an emergency situation. An educational intervention to improve water and sanitation behaviours (such as lack of handwashing before preparing food and during taking food, open defaecation by children in the family compound, inattention to proper disposal of garbage and faeces) resulted in prevention of diarrhoeal epidemics (PAHO 1982; Esrey *et al.* 1985).

References

- Anonymus (1978). Water with sugar and salt (Editorial). *Lancet* i i : 300.
- Bhattacharya S. K., Deb A. K., Nair G. B. (1999). Enteric Pathogens. In : National report (1994-1999) of the Indian National Committee of the International Union of Microbiological Society (IUMS). *Indian National Science Academy*. 227-246.
- Bhattacharya S. K., Bhattacharya M. K., Nair G. B., Dutta D. Deb A, Ramurthy T, *et al.* (1993). Clinical profile of acute diarrhoeal cases infected with new epidemic strains of *Vibrio cholerae* 0139 : Designation of the disease as cholera. *J Infect* 27 : 11-5.
- Bhattacharya S.K., Dutta P, Datta D, Bhattacharya M.K., Sen D, Saha M.R. *et al.* (1987). Relative efficacy of Trimethoprim-Sulphamethoxazole and nalidixic acid for acute invasive diarrhoea. *Antimicrob Agent Cemethor* 31 : 337.

- Bhattacharya S. K., Bhattacharya M. K., Dutta P, Sen D, Rasaily R, Moitra A, *et al.* (1991). Randomised clinical trial of norfloxacin for shigellosis. *Am J Trop Med Hyg* 45 : 683-7.
- Bhattacharya S. K., Bhattacharya M. K., Datta D, Dutta S, Deb M, Deb A, *et al.* (1997). Double blind, randomised clinical trial for safety and efficacy of norfloxacin for shigellosis in children. *Acta Pediatr* 86 : 319-20.
- Bhattacharya S. K., Bhattacharya M. K. , Dutta D, Mitra U, Dutta P, Dutta A,(1994). The rational use of drugs in the treatment of acute diarrhoea. *J Assoc Phys India* 42 : 503-5.
- Bennish M. L., Salam A. M., Haider R, Rarza M. (1990). Therapy for shigellosis. II. Randomised double blind comparison of ciprofloxacin and ampicillin. *J Infect Dis* 162 : 711-6.
- Cantey J. R. (1985). Infectious diarrhoea. Pathogenesis and risk factors. *Amer J Med* 78 (Suppl 68) : 65-75.
- Deb B. C., Sengupta P. G., Sircar B. K., Mondal S, Gupta D. N., Saha N. C., *et al.* (1985). Use of : Home available fluids" by mothers in the management of acute diarrhoea cases. *Third Asian Conference on Diarrhoeal Diseases*, Bangkok, pp. 242.
- Deb B. C., Sircar B. K., Sengupta P. G., De S. P., Mondal S, Gupta D. N., *et al.*(1986) Studies on intervention to prevent cholera transmission in urban slum. *Bull Wild Hlth Org* 64 : 127-31.
- Dutta P, Dutta D, Bhattacharya S. K., Datta A, Bhattacharya D. N. ,Pal S. C. (1984). Effectiveness of oral glucose electrolyte solution in the treatment of acute diarrhoea in neonates and young infants. *Indian J Med Res* 80 : 432-8.
- Dutta P, Bhattacharya S. K., Datta D, , Mitra U, Bhattacharya M. K., Rasaily R, *et al.* (1991). Oral rehydration solution containing 90 millimole sodium is safe and useful in treating diarrhoea in severely malnourished children. *J Diarr Dis Res* 9 : 118-22.
- Dutta P, Sen D. (1990). Outbreak dysentery due to nalidixic acid resistant *Shigella dysentery* type 1 at Agartala, Tripura : a hospital based study. *Indian J Pub Hlth* 34 : 38-40.
- De S, Chowdhuri A, Dutta P, Datta D, De S. P., Pal S. C. (1975). Doxycycline in the treatment of cholera. *Bull Wld Hlth Org* 54 : 177-9.
- Esrey S. A., Feechem R. G. and Hughes J. M. (1985). Intervention for the control of diarrhoeal diseases among young children : improving water supplies and excreta disposal facilities. *Bull Wld Hlth Org* 63 : 757-772.
- Formal S. B., Hale T. L., Boeleker E. C. (1983). Interactions on enteric pathogens and intestinal mucosa. *Phil Trans R Soc Lond* B 303: 65-73.
- Formal S. B., Hale T. L., Sansonetti P. J. (1983a). Invasive enteric pathogens. *Rev Infect Dis* 5 (Suppl-4) : S 702-7.

- Hirschhorn N, Kinzie J., Sachar D. B., Northrub R, Taylor J. O., Ahmed S, Phillips R. A. (1968). Decrease in net stool output in cholera during intestinal perfusion with glucose containing solution. *New Eng J Med* 279 : 176-81.
- Jalliffe D. B., Jelliffe E. F. P. (1981). Breast milk and infection. *Lancet* ii : 419.
- Karshner W. A., Curlin G. T., Huq M. I., Hirschhron N. (1970). Furazolidone in pediatric cholera. *Bull Word Hlth Org* 43 : 373-8.
- Khan M. C., Samidulla M (1982). Interruption of shigellosis by hand washing. *Trans Roy Soc Trop Med Hyg* 76 : 164-8.
- Mukherjee A. K., Garg S, Mitra R, Basu A, Rajendra K, Datta D, *et al.* (1996). Temporal shift in trait of *Vibrio cholerae* strains isolated from hospitalised patients in Calcutta : A 3 years (1993-1995) anaysis. *J Clin Microbiol* 34 : 2537-43.
- Manchanda V. K. (1996). Oral rehydration therapy programme in India; standard case management of acute diarrhoea. *J Indian Med Assoc* 93 : 220-6.
- National Child Survival and Safe Motherhood Programme (1994). New Delhi : Government of India, 79-85.
- Pizarro D, Pasada G, Lavine MM, Mohn E. (1980). Oral rehydration of infants with acute diarrhoeal dehydration : A practical method. *J Trop Med Hyg* 83 : 241-5.
- Pan American Health Organizations (1982). A guide to emergency health. Management after natural disaster. Scientific Publication No. 419.
- Registrar General, India. A Survey on Infant and Child mortality 1979. New Delhi; Ministry of Home Affairs.
- Sachar D. B., Taylor J. O., Saha J. B., Phillips R. A. (1965). International transmural electric potential and its response to glucose in acute and convalescent cholera. *Gastroenterol* 56 : 512-8.
- Salam M. A., Bennis M. L. (1988). Therpy for shigellosis. I. Randomised double blind trial of nalidixic acid in childhood shigellosis. *J. Pediatr* 113 : 901-7.
- WHO (1990). A manual for the treatment of diarrhoea for physicians and health workers. WHO/CDD/SER/80.2 Rev 2.

Chapter - 15
Development of Diagnostic for *Giardia lamblia*

S. Ghosh[1], A Sil[1], D J Chattopadhyay[1] and P Das[2]

Abstract

Giardia lamblia is an aerotolerant protozoan parasite that is common cause of human giardiasis. It inhabits the small intestine and causes diarrhoea with a diverge range of symptoms ranging from asymptomatic carrier stage to severe malabsorption, diarrhoea and weight loss. It is the most common diarrhoeal illness sometimes leading to epidemics. The management of the disease is made difficult by the availability of only insensitive and nonspecific diagnostic methods. Conventionally the diagnosis is made by microscopic examination of stool samples for the presence of cysts or trophozoites. Giardia cysts are shed sporadically and their number may vary from day to day. Routine examination of stool samples collected on consecutive days or even the recommended ten days time frame may mot confirm infection with this organism. Only 50% to 70% sensitivity has been reported by this technique. The low sensitivity is due to irregular excretion of cysts or trophozoites and examination of stool samples by unskilled personnel. We developed a PCR based assay to amplify and detect a segment of rDNA of G. lamblia and found it to be highly efficient in diagnosis of giardiasis.

Introduction

Giardia lamblia the gut protozoan parasite was first discovered by Anton Van Leeuwenhoek in 1681 from his own diarrhoic stool (Dobell, 1920). Little progress was made in investigation or description of the flagellate till 1859 when Lambl reported the

---

1. Dept. of Biochemistry & Dr. B C Guha Centre for Genetic Engineering and Biotechnology, University of Calcutta, 35 B.C. Road, Kolkata-700019.
2. Dept. of Microbiology, National Institute of Cholera and Enteric Diseases, ICMR, Kolkata-700010.

morphology in greater details (Lambl, 1859). Following this early investigation, there was a flurry of activity in the light microscopic description of *Giardia* (Fillice, 1952). A lack of agreement regarding nomenclature had existed from the time this organism was first described and still continues to be a subject of confusion. The nomenclatural problems involve both genus and species. The genus *Giardia* has been named by Kunstler in 1882 (Kunstler, 1882). However Blanchard in 1888 suggested that the genus be named *lamblia* in commemoration of the parasite's first accurate description by Lambl (Thompson *et al.*, 1990). It was Stites, who in 1915 (Stites, 1915) named this parasite as *Giardia lamblia.*

G. lamblia has two life cycle stages, the vegetative trophozoite stage and the infective cyst stage. Each of these stages is well adapted to survival in very different and hostile environments. The dormant quadrinucleate, ovoid cyst form that is responsible for transmission of giardiasis, persists in fresh water even at 4^0C (Bingham and Meyer, 1979). Infection normally follows ingestion of cysts in fecally contaminated water or less commonly via foods (Adam, 1991). After excystation, the emerging parasite quickly divides into two equivalent binucleate trophozoites that attaches and specifically colonize the human small intestine. They swim in the lumenal fluid with four pairs of flagella and also adhere to mucus strand *in vivo* and *in vitro* (Adam, 1991). They also penetrate the mucus layer to attach to intestinal epithelial cells via their unique ventral adhesive disc (Friend, 1966; Nemanic, 1979). In this position they feed on the content of the host gut not by phagocytosing large particles such as bacteria but through micropinocytotic vesicles. Here they multiply by binary fission. When the trophozoites are carried downstream by the flow of the intestinal fluid they encyst, as they could not survive outside the host.

G. lamblia is a major cause of waterborne enteric disease, giardiasis throughout the world (Nash, 1989; Wolfe, 1990; Adam, 1991). Millions of people worldwide is infected annually by this parasite (Warren, 1989). Morbidity is high, especially in children infected with *G. duodenalis* (synonymous with *G. lamblia* and *G. intestinalis),* the human parasite which recognizes no socio-economic, political or geographical boundaries (Boreham, 1991). The management of the disease is made difficult because of the unavailability of specific and sensitive diagnostic tool for the parasite. Conventionally the diagnosis is made by microscopic examination of stool samples for the presence of cysts or trophozoites (Goka *et al.*, 1990). *Giardia* cysts are shed sporadically and their number may vary from day to day (Garcia and Bruckner, 1997). Moreover despite symptoms some patients may not excrete cysts for several weeks. So routine examinations of stool specimens collected on consecutive days or even within the recommended ten days time frame may not confirm infection with this organism. Sampling over long periods of time may therefore be necessary (Danciger and Lopez, 1975; Hiatt *et al.*, 1995). These problems reduce the sensitivity of the method. Only 50% to 70% sensitivity has been reported by this technique (Bruke, 1997). Another reason for low sensitivity is the examination of stool samples by unskilled personnel (Danciger and Lopez, 1975). Other methods such as jejunal biopsy and duodenal aspirate examination gave better results but they find little utility, as they are invasive (Bown, *et al.*, 1996).

Immunological method of detection of the parasite based on detection of *Giardia* specific antibody in serum and antigens in the stool shows better result over conventional microscopy (Dedcova *et al.*, 1999). Diagnosis based on indirect immunofluorescence to detect *Giardia* cysts in stool samples using cyst-specific anti *Giardia lamblia* monoclonal antibody has also been reported (Winiecka-krusnell and Linder, 1995). Infact a number of immunoassay kits (enzyme immunoassay and direct flourescence) are available in the market for detection of *Giardia* in fecal specimens (Garcia and Shimizu, 1997). Though above 90% specificity and sensitivity has been claimed for detection of the parasite by these methods, determination of serum anti-*Giardia* antibodies has not been found satisfactory for the demonstration of giardiasis (Jokipii *et al.*, 1988). There is always chance of getting false results due to cross reactivity with other microorganisms.

In the last few years DNA based diagnosis of diseases is gaining importance. This system has the advantage over other diagnostic methods for being highly specific and at the same time sensitive as it relies on the sequence of the DNA. Moseley *et al.*, first reported the use of DNA probes to detect organisms harboring the genes encoding LT enterotoxins in enterotoxigenic *E. coli* in 1980 (Moseley *et al.*, 1980). Thereafter lots of DNA based diagnostic probes for detection of different pathogens have been reported (Ambinder *et al.*, 1985). Wirth and Pratt, were the first to demonstrate the utility of DNA probe for direct detection of parasitic agents in clinical lesions (Wirth and Pratt, 1982). A number of DNA-probe based diagnosis for giardiasis has also been reported. In 1989 Butcher reported a DNA probe for diagnosis of *Giardia* (Butcher and Farthing, 1989). In 1990 Lewis *et al.* reported total genomic DNA as probe which can detect as much as 10μg of *G. lamblia* DNA, 10^4 trophozoites and 10^4 cysts (Lewis *et al.*, 1990). But it showed cross reactivity with high amount (5μg) of *T. cruzi.*

The technique of gene amplification by polymerase chain reaction (PCR) (Saiki and Amhein, 1985) has revolutionized the field of molecular diagnosis because of its power to produce many copies ϱf a desired, previously undetectable nucleic acid target. PCR allows detection of organisms present in very low numbers by amplifying specific DNA segments in a few hours. This is a definite advantage over DNA-probe based diagnosis and people rapidly shifted over to PCR-based diagnosis. Within a span of few years number of reports came on PCR based diagnosis and epidemiological studies of different organisms. PCR has been used for the detection of bacterial, viral and protozoal pathogens. The first utilization of PCR in detection of *Giardia* from wastewater was done by Atlas who employed the giardin gene as the amplification target (Atlas, 1991). A 163bp region of heat shock protein (HSB) gene region of *Giardia* has also been employed in the detection of the parasite (Abbaszadegan *et al.*, 1993). Weiss was the first to report the PCR detection of the parasite from fecal specimen targeting a 183bp region of the SSU rRNA (Weiss, 1933). But all these methods required rigorous processing of water or clinical samples which often takes a day.

Ribosomal RNA gene is a very good target for amplification by PCR as it is present in higher copy numbers (Waters, and McCutchan, 1990). In *G. lamblia* there are about 63-132 copies of rRNA gene per nucleus arranged in tandem repeat (Boothroyd *et al.*, 1987; Sil, *et al.*, 1998). The present work is aimed at developing a PCR based assay to amplify and detect a segment of the IGS region of rRNA of *Giardia lamblia* which were found to be *Giardia* specific (Sil, *et al.*, 1998).

Materials and methods

Cultivation of *Giardia lamblia*

Two local isolates of *Giardia lamblia* and the reference Portland-1 strain (ATCC 30888) were routinely maintained in filter sterilised TYI-S-33 medium (Diamond *et al.* 1978) containing vitamin mixture and 10% heat inactivated bovine serum. The isolates were sub-cultured thrice a week.

Cultivation of other enteropathogens

Three different enteropathogens namely *Escherischia coli, Shigella dysenteriae* and *Entamoeba histolytica* were cultured in different media. Trophozoites of *E. histolytica* were grown in TYI-S-33 medium at 37^{0}C. *E. Coli* and *S. dysenteriae* were cultured at 37^{0}C in Tryptic Soy Broth.

Isolation of genomic DNAs

Giardia trophozoites (2 x 10^7) of late log phase were harvested by chilling the culture tubes on ice and then centrifuged at 600g for 10 min. The cell pellet was resuspended in 1ml of phosphate buffered saline (PBS). Nuclei from the cells were obtained by lysing the cells in 2 ml NP40 (Sigma chemicals, USA) solution (1% NP40 in PBS) followed by centrifugation at 500 g for 5 min. Subsequently nuclei were lysed by 2 ml of lysis buffer. The mixture was incubated overnight at 50^{0}C. The lysate was mixed with CTAB/NaCI solution and incubated at 65^{0}C for 10 min. Subsequently an equal volume of chloroform : isoamyl alcohol (24 : 1) was added, mixed gently and centrifuged for 5 min at room temperature. The aqueous phase was taken, extracted with equal volume of phenol : chloroform : isoamyl alcohol (25:24:1) and total nucleic acids were precipitated with 2.5 volume of absolute ehtanol containing 0.3M sodium acetate (pH-4.8). Contaminating RNA was removed by RNaseA digestion for 30 min at 37^{0}C. Thereafter the solution was extracted with phenol/chloroform/ethanol and then ethanol precipitated.

The procedure for isolation of genomic DNA from the other enteric pathogens was identical to that followed for DNA extraction from *Giardia* nuclei.

Isolation of plasmid DNA

Plasmid DNA was isolated using alkaline lysis protocol. 1.5 ml of overnight culture grown at 37^{0}C in LB, containing the appropriate antibiotic was pelleted at 4^{0}C. The pellet was resuspended in 100 μl solution I and kept in ice for 5 min. 200 μl freshly prepared solution II was added to this, mixed thoroughly by inversion and kept in ice for 5min. Then 150 μl 3M sodium acetate was added mixed properly and kept in ice again for another 5min. The mixture was then centrifuged at 12,000g for 15 min at 4^{0}C. The supernatant was carefully transferred to a fresh tube, RNase A was added to a final concentration of 2 mg/ml and the tube was incubated at 37^{0}C for 20min. To this equal volume of phenol : chloroform : isoamyl alcohol mixture (25:24:1) was added mixed by vortexing and the two phases were separated by centrifugation at 12,000g for 5 min. The aqueous phase was transferred to a fresh tube and plasmid DNA was precipitated by adding 2.5 volumes of absolute ethanol. The tube was kept at -20^{0}C for 30min to allow complete precipitation of DNA. Then the tube was centrifuged at 12,000g at 4^{0}C for 15min. Supernatant was discarded and the DNA pellet was washed with 70% ethanol, vacuum dried and suspended in 50 μl sterile water. The isolated DNA was estimated qualitatively by running a 0.8% agarose gel.

Southern Blot Hybridization

Approximately 3-10 μg of genomic DNAs of different enteropathogens were run on agarose gel and transferred on to a nytran membrane which was then baked at 80^{0}C for 2 h. The membrane was incubated for 4 h at 65^{0}C with prehybridization solution and then hybridized with different labeled IGS probes for 20 h at 68^{0}C. Subsequently the membrane was rinsed once with 5X SSC, 0.5% SDS at 65^{0}C for 5 min, twice with 0.1X SSC,1% SDS at 50^{0}C for 40 min and once with 2X SSC for 5 min at room temperature. The membrane was dried and exposed to X-ray flim.

Polymerase chain reaction

The PCR was carried out in 25 μl volume containing 5 μl of DNA extract or 1μl of the first PCR product. Reaction mixture contained 10 mM Tris-HCI (pH 9), 50 mM KCI, 1.5 mM $MgCI_2$, 0.01% gelatin, 250 μM deoxynucleotide triphosphate mix (dATP, dGTP, dCTP and dTTP), 3U of Taq Polymerase (Bangalore Genei) and 200ng of each primers. 30 cycles were performed for both reactions with denaturation at 95^{0}C for 60 seconds, annealing at 55^{0}C for 60 seconds and extension at 72^{0}C for 60 seconds. The reaction mixture was incubated initially at 95^{0}C for 5 min for complete denaturation of the template and at 72^{0}C for 5 min for final extension at the end of the reaction. Products of first PCR were visualized on a 1.5% agarose gel and for nested PCR in 2% agarose gel.

Results

Differentiation of *Giardia lamblia* from other enteric pathogens using intergenic NTS region as probe

The 5.6 Kb rRNA gene of the parasite has been cloned and restriction mapped (Sil *et al.*, 1998). The intergenic spacer (IGS) region represented by the 0.2kb BamHI-PstI, 0.3Kb PstI-PstI and 0.8Kb PstI-PstI fragments. In order to see whether this intergenic region could be used to distinguish *Giardia* from other enteric pathogens Southern blot was done using the above mentioned intergenic fragments as probes. It was found that the intergenic probes could differentiate *Giardia lamblia* from other enteric pathogens (data not shown) . Thus the intergenic region of rRNA gene of *Giardia lamblia* could be used as a target for diagnosis of the parasite.

Development of PCR based diagnosis for giardiasis

The intergenic region of the rRNA gene was sequenced and from the sequence two primers AS1 and AS2 were designed that would amplify a 550bp region of the IGS by PCR (Fig 1). The specificity of the primers were tested using genomic DNAs of different enteropathogens. The 550bp amplified product was obtained only for *G. lamblia* (data not shown). The primers could not differentiate between two strains of *Giardia* PD1 and PD2 but could differentiate between *Giardia* and three other enterpathogens. This was expected since the primers were derived from the intergenic regions of the rRNA gene of *Giardia lamblia* that is *Giardia* specific. The primers were found to be sensitive enough to detect as little as 2.5pg of plasmid DNA containing the rRNA gene and a minimum of 10 trophozoites. Taking the DNA content of one trophozoite to be 0.144pg (Erlandsen and Rasch, 1994) the reaction was sensitive enough to detect 1.44pg of *Giardia* genomic DNA.

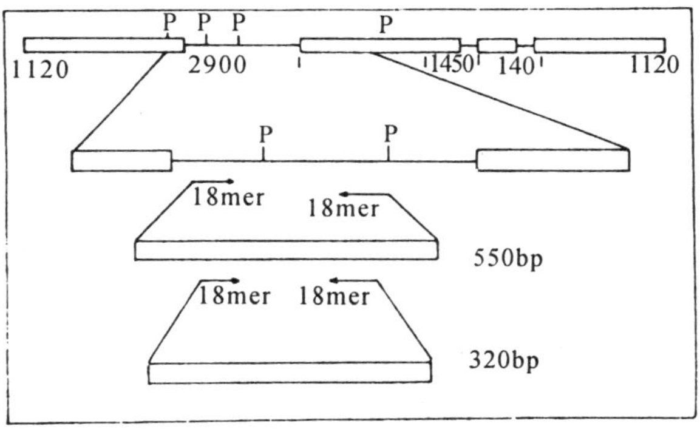

Fig 1. Amplification strategy from the intergenic spacer region (IGS) of multicopy rRNA gene of *Giardia lamblia* showing positions of primers. AS1 and AS2 amplifies a 552bp segment of the IGS. Primers SG3 and SG4 amplifies a 320bp fragment within the first PCR product. SS : small subunit ribosomal RNA; LS : subunit ribosomal RNA; P: PstI.

To assess the utility of the method for diagnosis, the assay system was employed on stool samples. This was initially investigated by using a model system similar to the one above, in which different dilution of cultivated *Giardia* trophozoites were added to a fecal specimen obtained from an adult with diarrhoea but microscopically negative of *Giardia*. Direct PCR of feces was known to be less sensitive than PCR of purified DNA because of the presence of inhibitory compound in stool like bilirubin, urobilinogens and the bile salts (Widjojoatmodjo *et al.*, 1992). One way of removal of inhibitiry substances was to purify the sample by treatment with a combination of detergent, protease and heat treatment (Weiss, 1933). But this procedure takes time and also adds expense to sample preparation that is disadvantageous when handling a lot of samples. Another way of overcoming the inhibitory effect was to do PCR in presence of bovine serum albumin (BSA) which has wide-spread use for relieving interference in PCR as well as in variety of enzymatic reactions (Hoss, *et al.*, 1992). But the easiest and cheapest way of removing the inhibition was by diluting the stool samples. This has been successfully utilized for detection of *Vibrio cholera* in stool samples (Varela, *et al.*, 1994). They had found that 100 times dilution of stool samples was sufficient to prevent inhibition of PCR reaction by contaminants. In our case the disadvantage of diluting the fecal specimen was that the number of *Giardia* parasite present in clinical sample was too low and there was every chance of diluting out the parasite or the DNA.

We tried different dilutions and found that fifty times dilution could relieve the inhibition. Different numbers of *Giardia* trophozoites were taken in 100 μl of control fecal sample that was found negative of *Giardia* and boiled for 10 min. It was then centrifuged at 12,000g. 20 μl of the supernatant was taken and diluted to 100 μl. From the diluted supernatant 5 μl was used for PCR amplification in 25 μl reaction. The entire PCR product was run in 1.5% agarose gel. It was observed that a minimum of 2000 trophozoites could be detected against a smeary background. In other word fifty times or more dilution of stool was optimal in minimizing the inhibition and specific amplification from 2000 trophozoites.

In reality it was not possible to get so many trophozoites in 100 μl stool. To increase the sensitivity nested PCR protocol was included in the assay. Nested primers SG3 and SG4 were designed that would amplify a 320bp region within the first PCR product. Different number of *Giardia* trophozoites were mixed with 100 μl of control stool specimen boiled 10 min and centrifuged at 12000g for 10 min. 20 μl of the supernatant was diluted to 200 μl and 5 μl of the diluted sample was subjected to PCR using primers AS1 and AS2 in a 25 μl reaction. 1 μl of the PCR product was subjected to nested PCR using primers SG3 and SG4. Inclusion of the nested PCR protocol increased the detection limit to 10 trophozoites if not less. The authencity of the 320bp nested PCR product was further checked by digesting the PCR product with PstI which yielded a 245bp fragment due to the presence of one PstI site in the amplified region of the rRNA (Fig. 2).

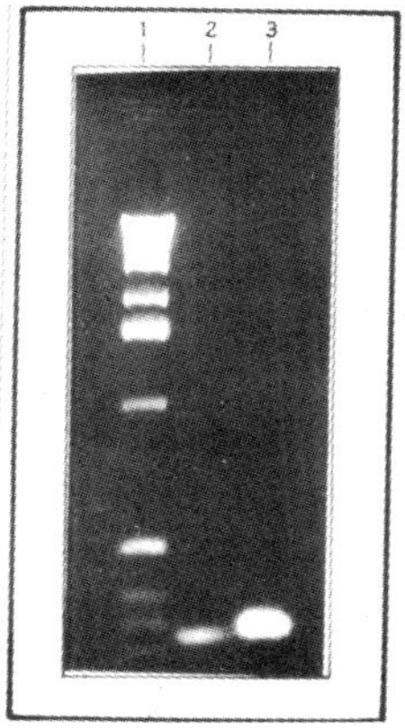

Fig 2. Confirmation of 320 bp amplified product by restriction digestion with PstI. Figure represents EtBr stained 2% agarose gel. Lane 1 : I kb DNA ladder; Lane 2 : 320 bp amplified product digested with PstI. Lane 3 : 320 bp amplified product.

Having tested the utility of our method we evaluated whether this method could be used to detect *Giardia* from clinical samples. 30 clinical samples reported to be positive for *Giardia* both by microscopy and immunological assays were subjected to PCR analysis followed by nested PCR. A 100% correlation was obtained with the other methods (Fig. 3).

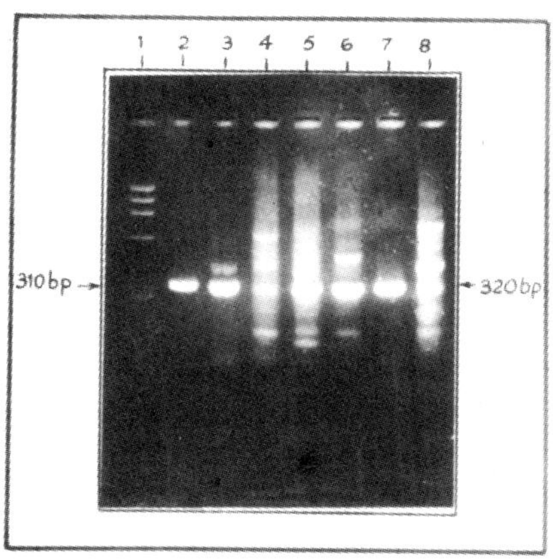

Fig 3. Detection of *Giardia lamblia* in clinical sample by nested PCR. Figure represents EtBr stained 2% agarose gel of 320bp nested PCR product. Lane 1: 0X174 HaeIII marker. The position of 310bp product shown by arrowhead. Lane 2 : positive control where amplification is obtained from plasmid containing rDNA. Lane 3 to 8 : amplification from different clinical samples that were tested positive of *Giardia* both by microscopy and immunological techniques.

Discussion

Accurate diagnosis of a disease is an important requirement for effective therapy. The diagnostic method should be highly sensitive, specific, reproducible, cost effective and also should not be time consuming. Conventionally, *Giardia lamblia* is diagnosed by microscopic examination of stool or by different immunoassays. Both the methods have their own limitations. Detection system based on DNA analysis successfully meets all the requirments for good diagnostic tools. Sensitive methods of nucleic acid detection have been devised for the specific detection of small amount of nucleic acid. The technique of gene amplification by polymerase chain reaction has revolutionized the fields of molecular biology because of its power to produce many copies of a desired, previously undetectable nucleic acid target. But before that, techniques must be devised for the amplification of microbial nucleic acid extracted from heterogenous human body fluids especially stool. Since there are many factors in stool that inhibits PCR reaction, methods that allow for nucleic acid amplification without substantial levels of inhibition or inconsistency must be devised. Also for obtaining best results a careful selection of primers for amplification of target molecule and extraction of template DNA has been suggested.

We have shown that the intergenic spacer region (IGS) of the rRNA gene of *G. lamblia* can be used as probe for identification of *G. lamblia* from other enteric pathogens (Sil *et al.*, 1998). In the present investigation primers designed from this region had been used for PCR detection of giardiasis. The primer pair AS1 and AS2 were found highly specific and sensitive in amplification of a 552bp region of the IGS because it didn't show any amplification from genomic DNAs of other enterpathogens and detected as little as 10 *Giardia* trophozoites. However the assay was not found so effective while amplification from stool samples. Different inhibitory substances present in stool hampered the PCR reaction. The inhibitory effect could be removed by extensive purification to generate PCR-compatible material. However, because purification adds to the time and expense of sample preparation, as well as to the loss of target nucleic acids, a more satisfying approach to the problem of PCR inhibition was to relieve the interference rather than attempt to remove all the offending substances. We chose to relieve the inhibition by dilution of the fecal sample. But this resulted in decreased sensitivity of the method. The sensitivity was restored by inclusion of the nested PCR protocol that amplified a 320bp region within the first PCR product. An added advantage of using the nested PCR steps was that it negated the chance of any false positive results in the first PCR that commonly observed during amplification from fecal samples. As a double check a PstI site was included in the amplified nested PCR product that indicate the uniqueness of the amplified DNA sequence. This type of follow up of the PCR product of specific size is needed when some controversy arises.

PCR-based diagnosis of giardiasis has been reported earlier targeting different genes of *G. lamblia*. Primers specific for *Giardia* targeted a 183-bp product from the small subunit (SSU) rRNA gene (Weiss, 1993); 218-and 171-bp amplicon from a giardin gene (Mahbubani *et al.*, 1992); and a 163-bp product from a heat shock protein (Abbaszadegan *et al.*, 1993) gene. An effective comparative study of these primers for detection of *G. lamblia* in water had been done (Rochelle *et al.*, 1997). The MAH433F-MAH592R primer pair that amplify 218-bp DNA from the giardin gene can distinguish between *G. lamblia* and *G. muris* but the sensitivity was very low and so a second round of PCR of 40 cycles with 5 µl of the product from the first reaction mixture was required. The ABB97F-ABB220R primer pair that amplifies a 163-bp DNA from heat shock protein gene gave amplification from both *G. lamblia* and *G. muris* though the amplification products differ considerably in size on the basis of which the two species could be distinguished. The WEI primer pair that amplifies a 183-bp product from the small subunit rRNA was found to give inefficient amplification of the correct-size product (183-bp) from purified cyst and no amplification from cysts seeded into environmental water samples. Moreover in addition to *G. lamblia* and *G. muris,* these primers also produced amplification products of various sizes from *Entaamoeba histolytica, Leishmania major* and *Trypanosoma brucei*. This may be because the primer targets the SSU rRNA gene that is known to have conserved sequences all along the evolutionary tree. Thus it was seen that none of the primer pair had the potential to meet all the requirements of a successful diagnostic tool.

In this respect our nested PCR method that target the IGS region of high copy number rDNA and is very specific for *Giardia lamblia* proved to be better than the previously mentioned PCR-based diagnostics. The nested PCR step helped in increasing the sensitivity and specificity of the method. The simplicity and cost effectiveness added to its advantage. Thus the highly sensitive nested PCR method is expected to contribute significantly in diagnosis of giardiasis.

References

- Abbaszadegan, M.; Huber, M. S.; Pepper, I. L. and Gerba, C. P.(1993). Detection of viable *Giardia* cysts in the water samples using polymerse chain reaction, pp. 529-548. In *Proceedings of the Water Quality Technology Conference,* American Water Works Association, Miami, Fla.
- Adam, R. D. (1991). The biology of *Giardia* Spp. *Microbiol. Rev. 55:* 706-732.
- Ambinder, R. E.; Wingard, J. R.; Burns, W. H.; Hayward, S. D.; Saral, R.; H. R.; Santos; Hayward, G. S. (1985). Detection of *Epstein-Barr* virus DNA in mouthwashes by hybridization. *J. Clin. Microbiol.* **21** : 353-356.
- Atlas, R. M. (1991). Environmental applications of the Polymerase chain Reaction. *ASM News.* **57**: 630-632.
- Bingham, A. K. and Meyer, E. A.(1979). *Giardia* excystation can be induced in *vitro* in acidic solutions. *Nature.* **277** : 301-2.
- Boothroyed, J. C.;Wang, A.; Campbell, D. A. and Wang, C. C. (1987). An unusually compact ribosomal DNA repeat in the protozoan *Giardia lamblia. Nucleic Acids Res.* **15** : 4065-4084.
- Boreham P. F. L. (1991). Giardiasis and its control. *Phar J.* **234 :** 271-274.
- Bruke, J. A.(1977). The clinical and laboratory diagnosis of giardiasis. *Crit. Rev. Clin. Lab. Sci.* **7 :** 373-391.
- Butcher, P.D. and Farthing, M. J. G. (1989). DNA probes for the fecal diagnosis of *Giardia lamblia* infections in man. *Biochem. Soc. Trans.* **17** : 363-364.
- Danciger, M. and Lopez, M. (1975). Number of *Giardia* in the feces of infected children. *Am. J. Trop. Med. Hyg.* **7 :** 237-242.
- Dedcova, L. M.; Volkov, G. N.; Serova, O. A.; Belanov, E. F.; Bormotov, N. I.; Krotova, V. A. and Ofitserov, V. I. (1999). The detection of antibodies to the trophozoite antigens of *Lamblia* by an immunoenzyme method. *Med. Parasitol (Mosk). Jan-Mar* **(1) :** 46-48.
- Diamond, L. S.; Harlow, D. R. and Cunnick, C. C. (1978). A new medium for the axenic cultivation of *Entamoeba histolytica* and other *Entamoeba. Trans. Roy Soc. Trop. Med. Hyg.* **72 :** 431-432.
- Dobell, C. (1920). The discovery of the intestinal protozoan of man. *Proc. R. Soc. Med.* **13 :** 175.
- Fillice, F. P. (1952). Studies on the cytology and life history of a *Giardia* from the laboratory rat. *Univ. Calif. Publ. Zool.* **57 :** 53-143.
- Friend, D. S. (1996). The fine structure of *Giardia muris. J. Cell Biol.* **29** : 317-32.

- Garcia, L. S. and Bruckner, D. A. (1997). *Diagnostic medical parasitology*, 3rd. ed., ASM Press, Washington, D. C.; National Committee for Clinical Laboratory Standards.
- Goka, A. K. G.; Rolston, D. D. K.; Mathan V. I. and Farthing, M. J. G. (1990). The relative merits of faecal and duodenal juice microscopy in the diagnosis of giardiasis. *Trans R. Soc. Trop. Med. Hyg.* **84** : 66-67.
- Hiatt, R. A.; Markell, E. K. and Ng, E. (1995). How many stool are necessary to detect pathogenic intestinal protozoa. *J. Trop. Med. Hyg.* **53 (1)** : 36-39.
- Hoss, M.; Kohn, M.; Paabo, S.; Knauer, F. and Scroder, W. (1992). Excrement analysis by PCR. *Science.* **359** : 199.
- Jokipii, L.; Miettinen, A. and Jokipii, A. M. M. (1988). Antibodies to cyst of *Giardia lamblia* in primary giardiasis and in the absense of giardiasis. *J. Clin. Microbiol.* **26** : 121-125.
- Kunstler, J. (1882). Sur Cinq, protozoires parasites nouveans. *Comptes Rendus des Seances dela Societe de Biologie et Ses Filiales.* **95** : 347-349.
- Lamble, W. (1859). Mikroskopische untersuchungen der Darm-Excrete. *Vierteljahrsch. Prakt. Heilkd.* **61** : 1-58.
- Mahbubani, M. H.; Bej, A. K.; Perlin, M. H.; Schaefer III, F. W.; Jakubowski, W. and Atlas, R. M. (1992). Differentiation of *Giardia duodenalis* from other *Giardia* spp. by using polymerase chain reaction and gene probes. *J. Clin. Microbiol.* **30** : 74-78.
- Moseley, S. I.; Echeverria, P.; Seriwatana, J.; Tirapat, C.; Chaicumpa, W.; Sakuldaipeara, T and Falkow, S. (1982). Identification of enterotoxigenic *E. coli* by colony hybridisation using three enterotoxin gene probes. *J. Infect. Dis.* **145** : 863-869.
- Nash, T. E. (1989). Antigenic variations in *Giardia lamblia. Experimental Parasitology.* **68** : 238-241.
- Nemanic, P. C.; Owen, R. L.; Stevens, D. P. and Mueller, J. C. (1979). Ultrastructural observations on giardiasis in a mouse model. II. Endosymbiosis and organelle distribution in *Giardia muris* and *Giardia lamblia. J. Infect. Dis.* **140** : 222-28.
- Rochelle, P. A.; De, L. R.; Stewart, M. H. and Wolfe, R. L. (1997). Comparison of primers and optimization of PCR conditions for detection of *Cryptosporidium parvum* and *Giardia lamblia* in water. *Appl. Environ. Microbiol.* **63 (1)** : 106-114.
- Saiki, A. K. and N. Arnheim, (1985). *Science.* **230** : 1350.
- Sil, A. K.; Das, P.; Bhattacharya, S.; Ghosh, S. and Chattopadhyay, D.J. (1988). Cloning of ribosomal RNA genes from an Indian isolate of *Giardia lamblia* and the use of intergenic nontranscribing spacer regions in differentiation of *Giardia* from other enteric pathogens. *J. Biosciences.* **23 (5)** : 557-564.

- Stites (1915). Cited from Creig., C. F. and Faust, E. C. (1970). *Chemical parasitology, 6th Rev.* Edn. By Faust, E.C.; Russel, P.F. and Jung, C.R.; Lea and Febiger Philadelphia, pp. 64.
- Varela, P.; Pollevick, G. D.; Rivas, M.; Chinen, I.; Binsztein, N.; Frasch, A. C. C. and Ugalde, R. A. (1994). Direct detection of *Vibrio cholerae* in stool samples. *J. Clin. Microbiol.* **32 (5)** : 1246-1248.
- Warren, K. S. (1989). Selective primary health care and parasitic diseases. In K. P. W. J. McAdam (ed.) : *New strategies in Parasitology.* New York: Churchill Livingstone, 217-231.
- Waters, A. P. and McCutchan, T. F. (1990). Ribosomal RNA : Nature's own Polymerase amplified target for diagnosis. *Parasitology Today.* **6 (2)** : 56-59.
- Weiss, J. B.(1993). PCR detection of *Giardia lamblia,* pp. 480-485. *In* D. H. Persing, T. F. smith, F. C. TEnover and T. J. White (ed.). *Diagnostic molecular microbiology : principals and applications.* American society for Microbiology, Washington, D. C.
- Weiss, J. B.; VanKeulen, H. and Nash, T. E. (1993). Classification of subgroups of *Giardia lamblia* based upon ribosomal RNA gene sequence using the Polymerase chain reaction. *Mol. Biochem Parasitol.* **54** : 73-86.
- Widjojoatmodjo, M. N., Fluit, A. C.; Torensma, R.; Verdonk, G. P. H. T. and Verhoef, J. (1992). The maganetic immuno polymerase chain reaction assey for direct detection of *salmonellae* in fecal samples. *J. Clin. Microbiol.* **30** : 3195-3199.
- Winiecka-Krusnell, J. and Linder, E. (1995). Detection of *Giardia lamblia* cysts in stool samples by immunofluorescence using monoclonal antibody. *Eur. J. Clin. Microbiol. Infect. Dis.* **14** : 218-222.
- Wirth, D. F. and Pratt, D. M. (1982). Rapid identification of *Leishmania* species by specific hybridisation of kinetoplast DNA in cutaneous lesions. *Proc. Natl. Acad. Sci. USA.* **79** : 6999-7003.
- Wolfe, M. S. (1990). Clinical symptoms and diagnosis by traditional methods. *In Giardiasis (Meyer E. D., ed),* pp. 175-185. Amsterdam : Elsevier.

Chapter - 16
Water Borne Diseases with a View to Hepatitis A and E Viruses Infection

*Prasanta Ranjan Bhattacharyya**

Abstract

Hepatitis A virus (HAV) and Hepatitis E virus (HEV) infections are the commonest causes of jaundice in developing and underdeveloped countries of the world within global distribution. In UK the incidence of HAV incidence rate is 15 per 1 million population. The sero-prevalence of HEV infection in Europe and USA is 1 to 2.5 compared to 10-15% in south east Asia. The preventive therapy for these two diseases are discussed in details in this paper.

Introduction

In ecology environmental health means the sum of conditions (including physical surroundings, climate and influence of other living organisms) which affect the health of human beings. Hepatitis A virus (HAV) and Hepatitis E virus (HEV) are such living organisms which affect the health of human beings through water and other means. Poor sanitation, sewage-contaminated drinking water, food, and milk, poor personal hygiene, overcrowding, and consumption of shell-fish grown in sewage-contaminated water propagate both HAV and HEV infections. Male homosex can also transmit both diseases (Mandal *et al.* 1999). Children are commonly affected by the HAV infection. Adults and children both are affected by the HEV infection in developing nations. Adults and elderly individuals in urban areas are prone to develop HAV infection even with good sanitation, improvement of personal hygiene, and education. Morbidity and mortality by

* Anandanibas, Ist Floor, Flat F&G, DE-3, Deshbandunagar, (North) Kolkata-700059.

HAV infection rises with age. High mortality is found with HEV infection in pregnancy (Mandal *et al.* 1999).

Epidemiology

HAV is one of the commonest cause of jaundice in developing and underdeveloped countries of the world. It is a global disease. Incidence of HAV infection is highest in children. Nearly 100% of children by the age of 5 years, and approximately 30% of adult population in USA are affected by HAV infection (Snyder & Pickering, 1996). 15 in 1 million population i.e. approx. 10,000 HAV cases per year are reported from UK. In developed nations 20% of young adults have serological evidence of past infection. 50 to 80% cases of jaundice due to acute viral hepatitis in India is from HAV infection. (Snyder and Pickering 1996). Anicteric infections are common in children with the ratio of 10:1, where as it is 1:1 in adults. (Mandal *et al.*, 1999)

HEV infection occurs sporadically in all countries, but epidemic occurs in developing nations. The seroprevalence of HEV infection in Europe and USA is 1-2.5%, as compared to 10-15% in South-East Asia. Outbreak of HEV infection occurred predominantly in the following countries e.g. South-East Asia, Burma, Nepal, former USSR, Mexico, Venezuela and North Africa due to gross sewage contamination of drinking water. There was an outbreak of HEV infection in Delhi in 1957, and 29,000 people were affected. Mortality rate in HEV infected pregnant women is very high, about 20-40%. (Mandal *et al.*, 1999).

Incubation period of HAV infection is 14 to 42 days, average 28 days, and of HEV infection is 14 to 63 days, average 42 days. Transmission of both diseases occurs faeco-orally through water. No carrier state develops and no vertical transmission occurs out of these two diseases. HAV and HEV infected individuals develop life long immunity after recovery from single attack.

Morphology of HAV & HEV

HAV belongs to the family of picorno virus, 27 nm, in diameter, RNA-enterovirus. HEV is a calici-virus and epidemiologically resembles HAV. (Mandal *et al.*, 1999)

Clinical manifestations of HAV & HEV infections

Distinction of HAV or HEV infections from other types of viral hepatitis on clinical ground is very difficult. Onset of HAV infection is gradual with low grade fever, myalgia, upper abdominal discomfort, anorexia, nausea and vomiting. 3 to 6 days after the above manifestations, urine becomes dark, faeces pale, and jaundice appears. Hepatomegaly is found nearly in all patients and splenomegaly in 20% of such patients. Adult smokers feel smoking distasteful. Arthralgia and rashes may also develop.

Clinical features of HEV infection is indistinguishable from HAV infection.

Complications of HAV & HEV infections

Complications of these two diseases are same.

(1) **Hepatic complications e.g.** (a) Fulminant hepatitis occurs in 0.1% cases with fatality rate of 20% in both diseases, but the fatality rate in HEV infected pregnant women rises upto 40%. The fatality rate also rises in HAV infected elderly individuals, (b) Cholestatic jaundice is a common problem but always resolves and remains benign. (c) Relapsing hepatitis develops 1 to 4 months after recovery associated with a return of hepatitis. but occurs rarely. (Mandal *et al.* 1999)

(2) **Extra-hepatic complications e.g.** (A) Aplastic anaemia, (b) Haemolytic anaemia, (c) Thrombocytopenia, and (d) Post hepatic syndrome (a Chronic fatigue syndrome).

Prognosis

HAV infection is usually a mild disease with fatality rate of 0.03% of patients under 55 years of age and 1.5% over 64 years of age. HEV is relatively a benign infection, besides high mortality in pregnancy from fulminant hepatic changes. (Mandal *et al.* 1999).

Therapy

(A) Curative therapy- There is no specific curative treatment of these two diseases. Bed rest and normal diet with no extra-fat is the mainstay treatment. In fulminant case, intensive care is necessary. Liver transplantation can be life saving. I.V. (intravenous) glucose 5-10% is good, but oral glucose therapy has got no scientific value. Sugar (5 ltsf), salt (5 pinches) in 8 oz.=200 ml.=2 teacupful water which must be boiled, then cooled, then it is to be served to drink with few drops of fresh lemon juice, 4-6 glasses daily. It would help to promote rapid recovery of jaundice. The scent of lemon helps to reduce the nausea and vomiting.

(B) Preventive therapy- It is important to control the spread of these diseases. Isolation of patients is not necessary. Spread of HAV or HEV infection can be controlled by good sanitation, supply of safe drinking water, good personal hygiene, avoiding over crowding, avoiding of food and water likely to be contaminated. Shellfishes should be cultured in sewage non-contaminated water to control the spread of these diseases.

Passive immunization (by normal immunoglobin 0.02 ml./Kg. body weight) is effective and provide protection for 3 months only.

It is necessary for travellers to endemic areas and also for exposure therapy[1,4].

Active immunization by anti-HAV vaccine is highly beneficial and it will also produce life long immunity against the HAV infection. No vaccine has yet been developed to prevent HEV infection. The recent development of highly immunogenic and safe formalin-killed vaccines marked a major advance in the prevention of HAV infection.

Anti-hepatitis virus A vaccine

This vaccine is now available in India, marketed by Smith-Kline-Beecham Pharmaceuticals (India) Ltd. The vaccine is named Havrix available in three strengths, 360, 720 (junior), and 1440 (adult). Havrix 360 is now available in combination with Hepatitis B vaccine. Havrix is a sterile suspension containing formaldehyde inactivated HAV (HM 175 Hepatitis A virus strain) absorbed on to Aluminium hydroxide. The virus is propagated in MRC 5 human diploid cells. It contained purified sterile suspension of inactivated HAV. The viral antigen content is determined by ELISA test. Havrix 720 junior and 1440 adult are standardised to ensure that the viral content is not less than 720 Elisa Unit in 0.5 ml. unit dose and 1440 Elisa Unit in 1.0 ml. unit dose. Havrix 720 junio is given to 1 to 18 years of age and 1440 adult is given to persons above 18 years of age. Two doses of this vaccine is given intramuscularly at an interval of 6 to 12 months, which gives immunity.

Diagnostic criteria for HAV & HEV infections

(A) **Non-specific** : Suspicion of hepatitis A will come from, (a) history of exposure, (b) very raised transaminases e.g. Alanine aminotransferase (ALT) or Aspartate aminotrans ferase (AST) above 1000 IU/liter., and (c) Prolonged prothrombin time (Satyasekaran M. 1999). A detailed clinical history and examination will suggest the diagnosis of HAV infection. Similarly, suspicion of hepatitis E will come from (a) history of recent arrival from HEV endemic area or travel to such area, (b) negative tests for HAV Igm antibody, HbsAg, and HCV antibody, (c) no risk factors for hepatitis B or C, and (d) no evidence of chronicity with return of LFT values to normal level (Mandal et al. 1999).

(B) **Confirmation** of HAV infection is done by HAV lgM antibody detection, which remains positive for first 12 weeks, then lgG antibody remains positive for life.

Confirmation of HEV infection by detection of lgM and lgG antibodies to HEV, HEV virus particles in stool by immune electron microscopy, and HEV-DNA by amplification through PCR (Polymerase chain reaction). None of the HEV specific investigations are routinely available at present (Mandal et al. 1999).

Discussion

Various official bodies around the world have recommended for use of hepatitis A virus vaccine. In USA, the Advisory Committee on Immunization Practices (ACIP) has recommended hepatitis A vaccination for high-risk groups e.g. (a) travellers to high endemicity areas, (b) homosexually active men. (c) children aged over 2 year living in high endemic areas, (d) illicit drug users and (e) persons with chronic liver diseases or clotting disorders. Hepatities A vaccine is a potentially powerful tool to control community-wide epidemics (Shaw, 1999). A community-wide outbreak of HAV infection occurred in Alaska in 1993. 5000 persons aged 1-34 years were vaccinated by Havrix in Alaska. The epidemic disappeared within 8 weeks in villages where 70-80% of the population were vaccinated, but the disease continued unabated where only 49% of the population were vaccinated (Shaw, 1999). Routine vaccination of children by Havrix has been introduced in some high-risk areas in USA. The ACIP has recommended routine hepatitis A vaccination to school children in 11 high-incidence states in USA (Shaw, 1999). The vaccine is recommended for risk groups e.g. travellers, sweage workers, and homosexuals in many European countries(Mandal, 1999). Prevalence of both disease has changed with improvement of personal hygiene, sanitation, living standard, education and safe drinking water supply. With less circulation of HAV, few incidence of Hepatitis A. Infection will develop and fewer children will be immune to this disease. There will be increased potential for hepatitis A infection in older children and adults. Risk of fatality rises with age (Snyder and Pierkering, 1996).

Prevalence Changes with Improvement of Hygiene

↓

Improvement in Sanitation and Living Standard

↓

Less Circulating Virus

↓

Fewer Incidence of Hepatitis A Fewer Children Becomes Immune

↓

Increased Potential for Hepatitis in Older Children and Adults

Hepatitis A : Clinical Characteristics of Patients by Age Group and Mortality Rate (Agarwal *et al.* 1999)

	Clinical Characteristics	Age in Years		
		<1-14 Yrs.	15-39 Yrs.	>40 Yrs.
1.	Jaundice	81.7%	86.8%	70.3%
2.	Hospitalized for Hepatitis	17.1%	23.2%	41.6%
3.	Death as a result of Hepatitis	0.1%	0.3%	2.1%

Common causes of viral hepatitis in India had been reported by WHO in a community of Rajasthan in 1997. The study reported the incidence of HAV 32.1%, HEV 7.1%, HBV 1.6%, HDV 3.8% and unclassified 55.4% (anonymous, 1997).

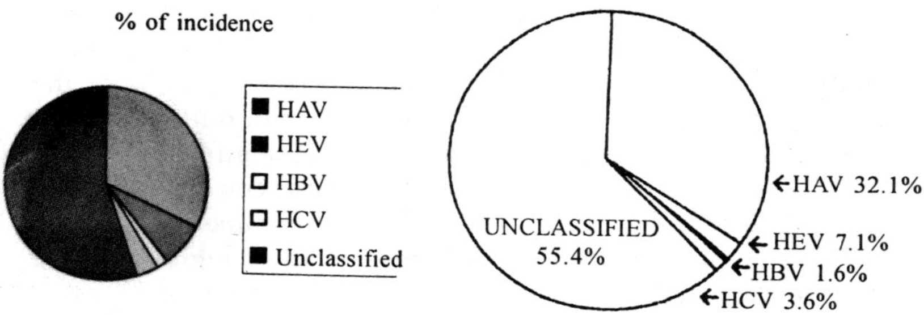

Fig. 1

A study conducted in Mumbai, where anti-HAV antibody was detected in only 77.5 % of children of the age group of 6-10 and 83.3% of the age group of 11-15 years respectively (Agarwal *et al.*, 1999). A recent study on the seroprevalence of antibodies to hepatitis A virus among children in Northern India by Rakesh *et al.* has shown that anti-HAV antibody prevalence in children increased with age, reached 96% by late childhood (Agarwal et al. 1999).

Prevalence rates of Antibodies of Hepatitis A Virus Among Healthy Children in Different Age Groups

Age Group in Yrs.	Number of Study Subjects	AntiHAVAntibody Positive Number (%)
0-5	28	19 (68%)
6-10	22	20 (91%)
11-18	23	22 (96%)

Socioeconomic condition has also got important effect on the incidence of HAV infection. Individuals belonging to middle and upper socio-economic strata, where anti-HAV antibody prevalence were 75% and 65% respectively, and in lower socioeconomic stratum were 78.8% and 91.3%.

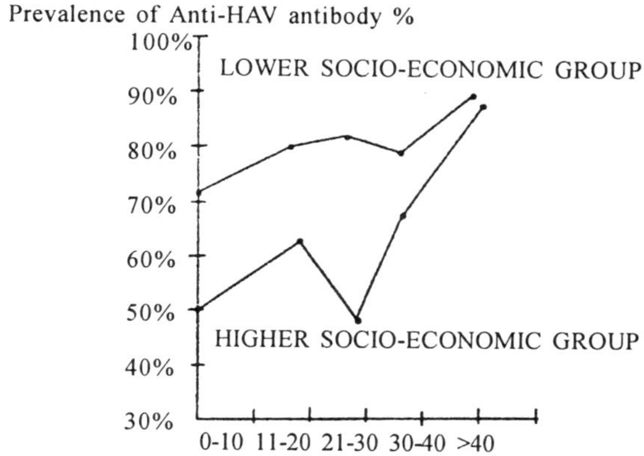

***Fig.* 2 Age Specific Prevalence of HAV in Comparison to Socioeconomic Group**

Similarly, in a study from Delhi, Anti-HAV antibody prevalence rate among 11-20 year old healthy subjects was only 39.8%. Anti-HAV antibody prevalence in persons with higher and lower socioeconomic status were 30.8% and 51.2% respectively. Based on such reports of relatively low anti-HAV antibody prevalence in young adults in India, it has been suggested that hepatitis A vaccination may be indicated in our population. Endemically the incidence of HAV infection is highest in children in comparison to higher age group of people (Agarwal et al. 1999).

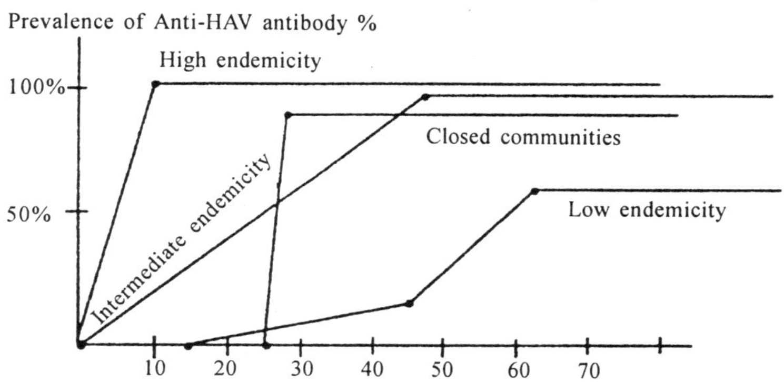

***Fig.* 3 Age Specific Prevalence of HAV in Accordance with Endemicity**

Conclusion

The people of higher socioeconomic group are conscious about their health, so they are less affected by these two diseases in early age. Immunity formation is delayed and the chances of infection by these diseases are more in older age with more complications and higher morality. Cost of anti-HAV vaccine is very high. It is now debatable whether the anti-HAV vaccine should be given compulsorily to all children or adults or it should be restricted to a particular socioeconomic group of people. In USA, many of its states are recommending this vaccine for routine immunization to children above one year of age, where epidemic prevalence is high. The incidence of HAV infection is 65-85% amongst all the cases of jaundice, reported from India (Agarwal et al. 1999). It would be advisable to introduce the anti-HAV vaccination for urban infants above one year of age from the middle and higher socioeconomic group of people who are at high risk.

References

- Agarwal R, Naik S, Yachha S K , Naik S R (1999) Seroprevalence antibodies to Hepatitis A virus among children in Northern India, *Indian Pediatr.* Vol. 36. No. 12 : pp. 1248-1250.
- Anonymous (1997) Common causes of Viral Hepatitis in Urban area of India: Community study in Rajasthan, *Bulletin of WHO*, OMS, 75.
- Mandal B K, Wilkins E C L, Dunbar E M, Mayon-White R T (1999) Lecture Notes on Infectious Diseases, Edn. 5th., published by Panthar Publishers Pvt. Ltd., Bangalore, India, pp. 216-396.
- Satyasekaran M (1999) Viral hepatitis, In IAP Text Book of Pediatrics, Eds. E Parthasarathi, P S N Menon, M K C Nair published by J. P. Brothers, New Delhi, pp. 393-396.
- Shaw F E (1999). The epidemiology and control of hepatitis A Vaccine: *Children & Practice*, 2. No. 1 pp. 5-7.
- Snyder John D and Pickering L K (1996) Hepatitis A through E, In: Nelson's Text Book of Pediatrics, Eds. Waldi E Nelson, Richard E Behrman, Robert M Kliegman, Ann M Arvin, Edn. 15th, published by W.B. Sunders, published by Prism Books Ltd., Banglore India, 1996: pg. 909-914.

Chapter - 17

A New Finding on Water Borne Disease 'Rhinosporidiosis' that Resolves Etiologic Controversies

Nidhi Maheshwari[1] *K B Ahluwalia*[2] *and R C Deka*[3]

Abstract

Rhinosporidiosis is a water borne disease endemic in some states of South India and very common in West Bengal. It is characterized by polypoid lesions in nose, nasopharynx, larynx, trachea, conjunctiva and a few other sites. Polyps of rhinosporidiosis are diagnosed histologically by presence of round bodies that resemble fungal sporangia filled with spores.

The etiological agent is believed to be the sporangium of a fungus Rhinosporidium seeberi whose life cycle could never be demonstrated outside the human host. Although the taxonomic position of R. seeberi remains inconclusive, most authors treat it as a fugus. Culture of this fungus as well as immunology tests have also been unsuccessful. Patients do not respond to anti-fungal nor other chemotherapies. Surgical extirpation and cauterization of the base of the lesion is the only form of treatment. After surgery, multiple recurrences are fairly common. Since the identity of the causal organism has remained doubtful, an effective form of treatment could not be developed. Several studies reporting contact of patients with pond/ lake water suggest that the etiological agent may be water borne.

In the present study samples of water from ponds and lakes used by patients in different endemic regions of India were analysed along with biopsies of nasal polyps. We have been able to isolate the cyanobacterium Microcystis aeruginosa from all the water samples. The bluish green

1. CIFE (ICAR), 30 GN block, Sector 4/5, Salt Lake, Kolkata- 700091.
2. Cell Biology and Electron Microscope Section, Dept. of Biophysics.
3. Department of Otolaryngology, AIIMS, New Delhi-110029.

cells of M. aeruginosa also have a colorless small cell stage called nanocyte which has been detected in clear waters of all the ponds and river samples studied. Both large cells and nanocytes of M. aeruginosa could be demonstrated inside the round bodies of rhinosporidiosis by light and electron microscopy. PCR using cyanaobacterial primers and universal bacterial primers (I6S rRNA) as well as fungal primers have indicated that spherules inside a round body belong to a cyanobacterium. Further work on sequencing the PCR product and formulation of drug therapy are in progress. It is hoped that if therapy becomes available, no surgery would be required for this disease.

Introduction

The etiology of rhinosporidiosis has been in dispute for almost hundred years (Guillermo Seeber, 1896 and 1900; O' Kinealy *et al.*, 1903; Ashworth, *et al.*, 1923; Vanbreuseghm, 1973; Thianprasit and Thagerngpol, 1989; Ahluwalia, 1992; Kennedy, 1995; Crissey, *et al.*, 1995 and Gaines, *et al.*, 1996). Polyps of rhinospridiosis contain microscopic round bodies that resemble fungal sporangia filled with spores. The sporangia are believed to belong to a fungus *Rhinosporidium seeberi*, the taxonomic position of which is doubtful and whose life cycle could never be demonstrated outside the human host (Ashworth, *et al.*, 1923; Jimenez, *et al.*, 1984; Thianprasit and Thagerngpol, 1989; Gaines, *et al.* 1996). Previous workers have also suggested that the organism may be protozoa (Seeber, 1900; O'Kinealy *et al.*, 1903), an alga (Vanbreuseghm, 1973) or an organism resembling the parasite of plant gall tumors (Crissey, *et al.*, 1995). The organism could neither be cultured in the laboratory, nor transmitted experimentally in animals (Thianprasit and Thagerngpol, 1989; Kennedy, 1995). Anti- fungal and other therapies are not effective. Surgical excision is not a cure and recurrences are seen fairly commonly. Electron microscopic studies in our laboratories demonstrated absence of any fungus in rhinospordoisis (Ahluwalia, 1992). The organism has been cultured successfully for the first time employing media generally used for cyanobacteria (Ahluwalia, 1999).

Case histories of patients showed the repeated bathing in natural waters of ponds and lakes, suggesting that the causal agent may be water borne (Thianprasit and Thagerngpol, 1989; Kennedy, 1995; Vukovic *et al.*, 1995). But samples of waters from ponds and lakes have not been analyzed. This study therefore, focusses on finding the causative organism in water samples of ponds, lakes and rivers in endemic regions in India, together with a parallel study on samples excised from polypoidal masses from clinically diagnosed patients of rhinosporidiosis.

Material and methods

Light, fluorescence confocal and electron microscopic methods standardised in our laboratory were used for study of biopsies, from patients coming to ENT department of All India Institute of Medical Sciences, New Delhi. Tissues were collected in sterile Tris buffer and fixed in 2% paraformaldehyde embedded in Durcupan and thin sections examined under EM. Paraffin sections were seen by light and confocal microscopies. The samples of natural waters from Bihar (Eastern India) and Mathura (North India), Trivandrum and Alleppey (South India) collected from exact locations where the patients were bathing , brought by relatives of the patients, were also examined under phase and fluorescence microscopes.

Two types of cells large blue green cells and small colourless nanocytes were isolated from water samples by centrifugation and processed for electron microscopy, immunocytochemical localization, and DNA studies. A detailed comparative study was carried out to determine whether both large cells and nanocytes of the cynaobacterium *M.aeruginosa* could be clearly recognised inside the round bodies of rhinosporidiosis by the following methods:

1. Light microscopic study using alcian blue, periodic acid Schiff (PAS), Feulgen and acridine orange staining.
2. Electron microscopy of round bodies of rhinosporidiosis and the organism obtained in natural water samples (Ahluwalia, 1992).
3. Antibodies (Polyclonal serum) was raised by injecting small and large cells (nanocyte and full grown stage) of *M. aeruginosa* and round bodies isolated from excised lesions in Tris buffer to three groups of caged mice, and tested by immunodiffusion (Ahluwalia *et al.*, 1997).
4. DNA extraction : DNA was extracted from a pure suspension of cells in pond water and from isolated intact round bodies in nasal polyps following the method of Porter (1988). Purity was checked by its ratio of A 260/ A 280.
5. Culture : Culture of isolated cells was done on organic medium consisting of sterile Tris buffer and glycerol (1:9) in presence of light at intensity of 2000 1x, and examined by phase contrast and fluorescence microscopy.

Results

Study of water samples : Two types of cell morphology (1) very small, colorless cells observed in clear water of all the natural water samples from Trivandrum, Allepey and Bihar and (2) the water bloom-like sample from the river bank in Mathura displayed clathrate colonies of a blue-green, large sized, single celled organism that was identified to be a cyanobacterium, *Microcystis aeruginosa*. The observed cells of *M. aeruginosa* were also confirmed by two different experts on Cyanobacteria. Among the large blue-green cells of *M. aeruginosa* the small single cells that had been observed in waters of Trivandrum, Alleppey and Bihar were also present. This small cell is actually a stage in the life cycle of *M. aeruginosa* and is termed as nanocyte and it is the main transmitting agent of the disease as it is present in apparently clear water and is invisible to naked eye.

Study of nasal polyps : Both stages of *M. aeruginosa* observed in natural waters were also recognised in sections of round bodies of rhinosporidiosis *in vivo.* Inside the round body the spherules are colourless, whereas in natural waters under sunlight, corresponding cells of *M. aeruginosa* contain bluish-green photosynthetic pigment. Interestingly, electron micrographs prepared from a very young lesion of rhinosporidiosis also showed multimellate photosynthetic vesicles with phycobilisome like structures inside round bodies similar to the pigment producing photosynthetic lamellae that are characteristic of *M. aeruginosa* cells growing in natural water under sunlight. These lamellae were absent in later stages of round bodies in clinical samples. Since the environment inside human epithelium is devoid of sunlight, the organism does not organize the photosynthetic apparatus consisting of lamellated vesicles with phycobilisomes and bluish green pigment. Subsequent observations on round bodies *in vivo* revealed all the stages of the cyanobacterium that had been found in natural waters studied by different methods as shown in table-1.

Table-1: Comparative Study of Cells Isolated from Water Samples and from Intact Round Bodies in Nasal Polyps

Methods	Observations on cells isolated from water samples		Observations on round bodies of nasal polyps	
Light microscopy	A very small (0.5 μm in diameter) colorless cell with dense, compact feulgen positive DNA, dispersed singly in clear water termed nanocyte and is a stage in the life cycle of cyanobacterium *Microcystis aeruginosa*	Ten times bigger than nanocyte, bluish- green cell with multiple inclusions organises clathrate colonies in water bloom-full grown stage *M. aeruginosa.*	Small, colorless spherules inside the round body and in form of linear fibrils	Round bodies originate from single cells of *M. aeruginosa* filled with multiple inclusions including refractile bodies.
Electron microscopy	Lack of discrete nucleus and internal organelles, wall structure contains peptidoglycan	Lack of nuclear membrane, and organelles, presence of photosynthetic lamellae	Lake of discrete nucleus, and organelles, wall structure contains peptidoglycan,	Presence of concentric multilamellate vesicles with phycobilisome like structures inside very young developing round bodies.
DNA extracted & Protein extracted	DNA extracted from *M. aeruginosa* in pond water showed 23 kb band; and protein extracted was cyanophycin.	Distinct band of 23kb when subjected to gel electrophoresis; cyanophycin in toluene showed by UV spectrophotometer absorbance at 628 nm was 0.106	DNA from *M. aeruginosa* inside the nasal polyps showed 23 kb band; and cyanophycin found in trace amount	23kb band shown on gel eletrophoresis cyanophycin present in nasal polyp was 0.002.
Polyclonal serum raised	No antibody detected		No antibody detected	
Culture	Grow on sterile glycerine under light of 2000 1 X intensity; some cells enlarge into round body like structures.	Grow on sterile glycerine under light of 2000 1 X intensity; some cells form round bodies.	Under continuous illumination the small cells were induced to become transformed into round bodies.	Induced round bodies acquired chlorophyll like blue-green pigment as well as concentric photosynthetic lamellae

The round body is nasal polyps is formed by enlargement of a single cell of *M. aeruginosa* and concomitant secretion of polysaccharide that assembles into linear fibrils that are added to the wall of the round body. Repeated multiplication gives rise to a large number of daughter *M. aeruginosa* cells inside the enlarging round bodies. During maturation the individual daughter cells of *M. aeruginosa* are also been to be enveloped by polysaccharide fibrils. At maturity numerous single celled organisms belonging to the two morphological forms of *M. aeruginosa* are liberated through pores in the wall of round body.

Culture of colonies of *M. aeroginosa* isolated from river water onto cavity slides with organic medium and by given 2000 1x of fluorescent white light showed in 3 days a few cells of *M. aeruginosa* enlarged and differentiated into round bodies almost similar to the round body in nasal lesions *in vivo*. The induced round bodies were initially colourless but after a span of illumination developed blue-green pigment. These observations suggested a link between *M.aeruginosa* in natural water and the round body in rhinosporidiosis. Autofluorescence was shown by only mature round bodies in unstained sections under ultraviolet excitation with 540 nm, whereas not by younger bodies. *M. aeruginosa* cells in natural waters did not show autofluorescence. Polyclonal serum bled from mice given *M. aeruginosa* from natural waters did not show any antibody raised against antigen from homogenate of round bodies *in vivo* as it gave weak reaction in immunodiffusion wells. Labelling of sections of polyps with the antibody in polyclonal serum and protein A-gold conjugates did not give conclusive results.

The round bodies *in vivo* display the distinctive features such as multiple inclusions, small nanocyte cells, linear fibrils, very mature refractile cells and autofluorescence in mature round bodies. Except autofluorescence, these features were also observed in colonies of *M. aerugoinosa* in natural water except autofluorescence.

Discussion

The comparative light and electron microscopic study demonstrates similarties between developmental stages of round bodies in nasal polyps and single celled cyanobacterium-*M.aeruginosa* isolated from pond waters where patients were bathing in different endemic regions of India. *M. aeruginosa* is a common cyanobacterium in water blooms found in nutrient rich fresh and brackish waters in tropical and temperate countries.

(Carr and Whitton, 1982). Animals that have been reported to develop rhinosporidiosis (Kennedy *et al.*, 1995; Moses and Balachandran, 1987; Allision *et al.*, 1986; Jimenez *et.al.*, 1986), could possibly have come in contact with water containing *M. aeruginosa*. In case of human beings the small-celled colorless nanocyte stage of *M.aeruginosa,* the transmitting agent of the disease detected in clear waters of Alleppey, Trivendrum, Bihar and Mathura could possibly enter human host through the nose. This study has demonstrated nanocytes in all the water samples analyzed as well as in round bodies in the excised nasal rhinosporidiosis masses. Thus, apparently clean waters from ponds and lakes and municipal and recreational waters need to be checked for the presence of colourless nanocyte stage of *M. aeruginosa*. Observations in culture showing transformation of *M. aeruginosa* cells from pond water in organic medium into round bodies lends additional support to *M. aeruginosa* as the causative organism of rhinosporidiosis.

The present work provides strong evidence that the spherules in round bodies in nasal rhinosporidiosis represent the unicellular cyanobacterium *Microcystis aeruginosa*. Although there is a superficial resemblence with fungal spores, there is no evidence of fungus in this disease. Cyanobacterias are prokaryotes characterized by absence of nuclear membrane, presence of peptidoglycan in cell wall, multiple cell inclusions as well as the proteinaceous cyanophycin granules, gas vacuoles and multilamellate vesicles. They divide by fission not by mitosis. Lamellated bodies have been observed by other workers (Kennedy *et al.*, 1995; Thianprasit and Thagerngpol, 1989; Apple, 1983), but their nature was not understood. It was only after study of natural water samples that our attention was drawn toward this aspect of the organism *in vivo*. The name rhinosporidiosis was originally given on the basis of fungal etiology (Ashworth, 1903). The findings of this study warrant a change of the name of this disease. Earlier we had suggested that starch from dietary tapioca that is consumed in endemic regions could become a possible source of polysaccharide for the wall of round body (Ahluwalia *et al.*, 1994). However, the present study has refuted that observation as it indicates that the polysaccharide in wall of round body is secreted by the unicelled Microcystis itself, and it does not come from an external source, earlier thought to be tapioca. Furthermore, the bodies inside spherules that were earlier interpreted as residue-loaded vesicles (Ahluwalia, 1992) are now found to be multiple inclusions that are characteristic of cyanobacteria (Carr and Whitton, 1982).

PCR using cyanaobacterial primers and universal bacterial primers (i6S rRNA) and fungal primers have also shown that the organism is a cyanobacterium. Further work on sequencing the PCR product and evaluation for drug therapy, using laboratory culture of the organism are in progress. It is hoped that if therapy becomes available, no surgery would be required for this disease.

Acknowledgement

Thanks are due to Dr. S. K. Kacker, former Professor of Otolaryngology, AIIMS, New Delhi, for suggesting this problem and to Dr. Manoj Raje, Scientist, Institute of Microbial Technology, Chandigarh, for useful discussion, D. K. Bassi, Technician, AIIMS provided techincal help. This work was supported by funds from All India Institute of Medical Sciences, CSIR & DST, Government of India.

References

- Ahluwalia K. B. (1992). New interpretations in rhinosporidiosis, entgmatic disease of the last nine decades, *J Submicroscop Cytol Pathol* **24** : 109-114.
- Ahluwalia K. B., Sharma N., Deka R. C., Kacker S. K. (1994). Association of tapioca and chronic inflammation with rhinosporidiosis. *Ind J Otolaryngol* **13** : 25-27.
- Ahluwalia K.B., Maheshwari N., Deka R.C (1997). Rhinosporidiosis : A study that resolves etiologic controversies. *Amer. J. Rhinology* **11** : 479-483.
- Allison, N., Willard, M. D., Bentic-Smith, J. & Devis, K (1986). Nasal rhinosporidiosis in two dogs. *J. Amer. Vet. Med. Assoc.* **188 (8)** : 869-871.
- Apple (1983). D. J. Papillome' der conjuncktiva bedingt durch Rhinosporidiose. Fortschr. *Ophthalmol.* **79** : 571-574.
- Ashworth J. H. (1923). On Rhinosporidium seeberi Wernike 1903, with special reference to its sporulation and affinities. *Trans Roy Soc Edinburgh* **53** : 301-342.
- Carr N. G., Whitton B. A. (1995). The Biology of Cyanobacteria. Oxford : Blackwell Scientific, 1982.
- Crissey J. T., Lang H, Parish L. C. Manual of Medical Mycology. Oxford: Blackwell Scientific, pp. 203-205.
- Gaines J. J., Clay J. R., Chandler F. W., *et al.* (1996). Rhinosporidiosis: Three domestic cases. *S Med J* **89** : 65-67.

- Jimenez, J. F. Young, D. E., Houngh, A. J. Jr. (1984). Rhinosporidiosis : a report of two cases from Arkansas. *Amer. J. Clin. Pathol.* **83 (5)** : 611-615.
- Kennedy F. A., Buggage R. R., Ajello L. Rhinosporidiosis (1995). A description of an unprecedented outbreak in captive swans (Cygnuc spp) and a proposal for reversion of the ontogenic nomenclature of *Rhinosporidium seeberi. J Med Vet Mycol* **33** : 157-165.
- Moses, J. S. & Balchandran, C. (1987). Rhinosporidiosis in bovines of Kanyakumari district, Tamil Nadu, India. *Mycopathologia* **100** (1) : 23-26.
- O'Kinealy F. (1903). Localised Psorospermosis of the mucous membrane of Theseptum nasi. *Proc Laryngol Soc Lond* **X** : 109-111.
- Porter, R. D. (1998).DNA transformation. *Methods in Enzymology.* **167** : 703-712.
- Seeber G. R. Un nuevo esporozoario parasito del hombre dos casos encontrados en polipos nasales. Thesis University nac de Buenos Aires, 1900.
- Thianprasit M, Thagerngpol K. (1989). Rhinosporidiosis. *Curr Topics Med Mycol* **3** : 64-85.
- Vanbreuseghm R. (1973). Ultrastructure of *Rhinosporidium seeberi. Int J Dermatol* **12** : 20-28.
- Vukovic Z, Bobic-Radovanovic A, Latkovic Z, Radovanovic Z (1995). An epideiological investigation of the first outbreak of rhinosporidiosis in Europe. *J Trop Med Hyg* **98** : 333-337.

Chapter - 18

Socio-Economic Aspect of Vector-Borne and Water-Borne Diseases

*Tapasi Biswas**

Abstract

That health conditions are positively correlated with income and level of living in a country, very few people in India can escape from being afflicted either chronically or intermittently with intestinal infection from water-borne diseases. Whatever the shortcomings in design and structure of the health administration in India, its basic weaknesses are those of insufficient funds, a scarcity of competent personnel, and an inadequate number of clinics, and hospitals. Administrative reforms cannot compensate for the poverty of national health facilities. Actually the mass campaign against these diseases will take place within a physical, social and economic framework which is generally less conducive to good health in India than in the advanced countries. There should be need for improved health legislation and more adequate law enforcement, ideally such policy measures in the legal and administrative fields should be integrated with the health campaigns, supporting them by providing inducements and punishments.

Introduction

Health conditions are intimately linked with almost every aspect of life in a society. The fact that improved health has an independent value for individual implies that the health facilities available are an important item in a country's standard of living. At the same time the availability of almost every other items of consumption, including foodstuffs, housing, clothing, sanitation, and

* Dept. of Economics, Vivekananda College, Kolkata

educational facilities, profoundly influence the health conditions. It is therefore natural to assume that health condition is positively correlated with income and level of living in a country, because more prosperous the people are, the better they are able to combat diseases and obtain adequate medical treatment. In spite of this, the higher income strata often fall prey to the vector-transmissible and water-borne diseases in India, for example, the recent outbreak of malaria in Kolkata's high-income locality. Very few people in India can escape from being afflicted either chronically or intermittently with intestinal infection from water like typhoid, dysentry, and diarrhoea. We find poverty in economic and cultural senses to be the primary cause of conditions that menace health though at the same time, inferior health conditions help to preserve poverty by lowering labour input and efficiency.

Historical accounts

The scanty historical accounts, which are available, indicate that leprosy, cholera, smallpox, malaria and intestinal worms have menaced Indian people since antiquity. Vector-borne diseases like malaria in this sense are indigenous. Before the post-war era, virtually everyone in South Asia was suffering in some manner from malaria. The disease was so common that it was responsible for from 5 to 20 percent of all deaths. With the introduction of DDT spraying, the situation has changed radically. In India, where about half the population lived in a highly malarious areas, large-scale control operations were started in 1953, as a result of which number of cases per year declined. Towards the end of the 1960's, malaria is expected to become so infrequent that the supervision of the work can be left entirely to local authorities (Myrdal, 1968). The government of India hoped that by the end of 1972, the entire population would be free of the disease. But the recent nearly epidemic condition of malaria in Kolkata shows that even with medical advancement we could not eradicate it totally. The problem with insect-borne disease is that bearer are the insects who are reservoir of the diseases unlike smallpox where bearer are human being. So vector-borne diseases create more problem of public health than the ordinary diseases.

Socio-economic aspect in urban and rural areas

The problem of rural and urban areas are different in this respect. In urban area, people are relatively more affluent and more conscious about their individual health. In spite of this, the problems are created by overcrowding, slum-dwellers, migrant laborers and other marginal people. They are the potential reservoir of these diseases. The resurgence of malaria in Kolkata shows that all these poverty -stricken people are the permanent source of infection. Because of the socio-economic problem, the richer are not spared from the epidemic though they can afford the treatment. This is the classical example of individual health problem in the midst of community health problem. The report on *'The Statesman'* on October, 22nd, 2000 "City hospital lacks drugs to fight Kala-azar" has shown that in The School of Tropical Medicine, about 30 Kala-azar patients were admitted till August, this year. Though the tropical disease was virtually eradicated in the country, we find an alarming number of Kala-azar cases from Bihar. Thus it can be speculated that Bihar migrant labourers whose number is large in comparison to labourers from other states have transmitted Kala-azar in Kolkata. Migrant labours cannot maintain the quality of life needed regarding health and hygiene. So they easily fall prey and act as the potential threat to the city dwellers.

In rural area, vector-borne disease like malaria generally attacks at planting and harvesting times, when hard labour is most needed and when food tends to be most scarce. Sometimes children of the family come to work to substitute their ill parents. Because of epidemic, labourers themselves become non-productive and ineffective. In this way society's valuable human resources get exhausted.

Water-borne disease occur due to sewerage disposal problem and contamination of water. The high rate of infant mortality is partly due to the prevalence of diarrhoea and other water-borne diseases. Aside from cholera, diseases in this category are rarely fatal except in early childhood (Harrison, 2001). Their principal threat is that they sap the vitality of their victims and adversely affect labor input and efficiency. For many of these diseases including typhoid fever, the new medical technology offers both cures and vaccines or other preventive agents. But as the latter are usually effective only for short periods, mass inoculations serve little purpose. Stamp out of these diseases will be very much easier if there are safe drinking water supply and good sewerage and drainage system and higher level of personal hygiene.

In urban area, haphazard growth of settlements without proper drainage system makes chaotic condition to the city dwellers. Example is the recent water logging in Kolkata. Sometimes drinking water supply is contaminated by old or unscientific sewerage system making epidemic in an area. Arsenic contamination of aquasphere of the underground water reservoir makes the problem worse. Actually in the urban area water supply and sewerage system are very complicated and vulnerable to any sort of endemic and epidemic. Slum-dwellings and continuous inflow of labor create pressure on the already over-burdened existing sewerage and safe water supply systems. Though higher income group somehow manages to keep away water-borne diseases by maintaining personal hygiene, lower income group, especially, children very often fell prey to these killer diseases. In rural areas problem is more or less same. The situation in rural West Bengal though improved much by supply of pure drinking water, there are some drought prone areas which suffer periodically. These are Purulia, parts of Bankura and Bardhaman (Mukherjee, 1999). It is found that, in rural area, not only drinking water to be made safer, water for other uses will be supplied safe to eradicate these water-borne diseases.

Compared to cities, in villages, there is scarce private facility. So the rural people have to depend fully on public health facilities available (Mukherjee, 1999). In urban area there is much scope to spend on private health care system. Thus it seems that the rich can be spared. But in case of vector-transmitted and communicable diseases, private health facility fails to protect even the richer. Here the problem is poverty in the midst of plenty. Since this community health problem does not create immediate disaster like food and drought, they are often overlooked.

Housing standards are abominably low in the city slums and rural districts. Overcrowding, together with inadequate sleeping arrangements, abets the spread of transmissible diseases. Sanitary conditions constitute a major health problems. The very low level of public sanitation has restricted the effectiveness of mass campaigns, particularly with regard to cholera and other water-borne diseases. Efforts are needed to provide pure water, effective sewerage systems and latrines in various localities. Very few people have the source of safe water supply. In rural areas the position is worse where safe water is more scarce.

Private and public expenditure

When diseases attack people in a locality, severe resource drainage occurs in both public and private sphere. Rich families can bear the cost of private medical services. Poor families at first try to combat diseases with their own meagre resource, but when this becomes out of their control they try to take help from outside agencies specially government medical services. In this way treatment becomes haphazard and irregular rather than consistent which makes problem more complicated, may be the loss of life. This, also creates a pressure on government hospitals, clinics as well as funds. On the other hand when this over-tolerant public health system becomes over-flooded with these patients, conditions become chaotic, creating multiple problems on the existing over-burdened system. With limited resources, treatment becomes inadequate and patient's sufferings become intolerable (Mukherjee, 1999). Just at the moment, because of sensational news spread by the media some emergency measures are undertaken by the government without any previous planning which becomes wastage after the end of the epidemic.

The two parts of mitigating the problem, preventive and curative can be looked on two levels, individual and community. In India about 40 percent people are living below the poverty line. So it is unexpected that they can take responsibility of their own health. Though NSS data has shown that even in the poorest rural communities, 2 to 3 percent of private income goes for drugs and medical care. It is likely that private expenditure exceeds the public expenditure and when both types of expenditure are added, spending on health services for the masses of people amounts to 3 to 5 percent of GNP (Myrdal 1968).

A minor part of the cost of health services in India is financed by foreign aid. Though the contributions of outside agencies cannot cover costs that the country himself will otherwise cover, but they are important in encouraging greater national efforts in the health field, which most often implies higher public expenditure.

Preventive part is more important than the curative part. Only after the improvements in sanitation and hygiene, curative measure will be effective. Though effective and inexpensive medications are available for the treatment of these diseases, since the source of infection are always present the medicinal treatments become ineffective. The efforts to prevent and cure will increasingly require reforms in the fields of nutrition, sanitation and hygiene and an increase in the supply of properly trained medical and paramedical personnel, equipments clinics and hospitals. All these are directly related with economic well being, health education and the social consciousness of people of the country.

Medical technology will be helpful, but mainly in conjunction with larger inputs in these other fields. Rapid development of the technology of preventive medicine economizes the utilization of skilled medical personnel by restricting their work to the planning and directing of functions. Though it would leave much of the fieldwork such as DDT spraying, the constructions of wells, drains and lavatories, and even the teaching of elementary hygiene for rural people and persons with little or no medical training.

About curative aspect, it can be said that regular orientation program of government physicians in private medical institution will update their knowledge about medical science. Government should take initiative for running Refreshers Courses for the doctors about advanced medical treatment available in the Western advanced countries. Though it requies public expenditure, its effects would be far reaching in comparison to measures undertaken during epidemic without a prior arrangements.

An important aspect of the preventive measures is the sound health intelligence system (Health Intelligence, 1991). If there is close network of intelligence system as in the advanced countries, the sources of contact will be immediately come to the notice of the authority and prompt measure can be undertaken before any epidemic occurs. Like doctors of Western advanced countries, if our doctors practice the preventive measures (DDT spraying) on their own they can realize the ground reality associated with these works and rectify the shortcomings of this work quickly.

Health monitoring system in West Bengal villages

Due to implementation of Multipurpose Health Worker System in West Bengal three tiers of workers are engaged in this work. 1. Female and male health workers at the grass root level 2. Female and male health supervisors in the middle tier and 3. Sanitory inspectors in the controlling tier (Mukherjee, 1999). All these workers have specific area of work. In addition to this, government of W.B. rested the responsibility of rural health monitoring on Panchayet so that people's representatives can determine work progress. There is permanent public health committee at block level who are supposed to know the health problem and take immediate measures of any sort of preventive, developmental, epidemic and emergency public health problem of the block. This permanent public health committee comprises members of the Panchayet, Block Medical Officer of Health, Public Health Nurse, Block Sanitary Inspector and the representatives of Block Development Officer.

Health administration in India

In India, most matters related to health come under the jurisdiction of the states. Because the states have not always be amenable to advise, the Central Council of health, which was established in 1952, and is composed if the health ministers of states, has not succeeded in coordinating India's health policies to the extent desirable (Myrdal, 1968). Urban areas are in a more or less autonomous position in regard to health matters. In India curative and preventive health services have been integrated at the top administrative level but not at the grassroot level except in a couple of states. Even where local health centers are designed to provide integrated health services, they often fall in this task because their personnel is insufficiently and inadequately trained in the methods of preventive medicine and because the burden of curative work is overwhelming.

Whatever the shortcomings in design and structure of the health administration in India, its basic weaknesses are those of insufficient funds, a scarcity of competent personnel, and an inadequate number of clinics and hospitals. Administrative reforms cannot compensate for the poverty of national health facilities.

Health legislation

Although many laws have been passed, the present body of health legislation is inadequate. Regulations are lacking on many vital subjects, for example, sanitary conditions are poorly regulated.

Health and five year plans

It is surprising that health programs have not so far given a high priority in the development plans of our country. Improved hygiene is rarely mentioned among the principal objectives of plans. Actually expenditure on health does not include expenditure on sanitation sewerage which is essential for the prevention of all these diseases.

From the planning point of view, the effect of any particular policy measure in the health fields depends on all other policy measures and is, by itself indeterminate. This means that it is impossible to impute any single measure or a set of measures to a definite return in terms of improved health conditions.

In India, about a third of the total sum allotted to health in the successive development plans is earmarked for water supply and sanitation sahemes. But accomplishment fell short of expectation because the work was poorly organized and skilled personnel and materials were lacking.

Conclusion

Actually the mass campaign against these diseases will took place within a physical, the social and economic framework which is generally less conducive to good health in India than in the advanced countries. Improved medical facilities, better sanitation and hygiene, all depend on economic level of a country. Both medical and educational facilities influence health condition. The improvements of public hygiene is not merely a problem of acquiring the necessary financial, material and human resources, it is also a problem of educating the masses. People must be taught to be more rational and more concerned about their health. Not only public hygiene but private hygiene is also important. The most elementary rule of health is personal cleanliness, though this is difficult to achieve when public sanitation is inadequate. Gandhi thus said that we must learn science of municipal sanitation from the west. He believed that " basic education" should include " the elementry principle of sanitation, hygiene and nutrition". Though maintenance of public hygiene is made through community development programme in some cases, private hygiene is still neglected in India. The fact is that scientific attitudes towards personal and public hygiene are interwoven into the very fabric of society (this include not only levels of living, literacy and education, but also social stratification, sexual mores, religious taboos and rites, and superstitious ideas about how diseases caused and transmitted) it does not imply that campaigns to improve habit of hygiene are hopeless. Teachers and schools should be more involved in this task. Education and the spread of more rational attitudes have a general bearing on health status that adds weight to all other reasons for adopting policies to improve education.

The task of instructing people about specific health hazards belongs more specifically to the health authorities, as does the task of improving sanitation. There should be need for improved health legislation and more adequate law enforcement. Ideally such policy measures in the legal and administrative fields should be integrated with the health campaigns, supported by providing inducements and punishments.

Further progress will increasingly depend on advances in popular co-operation, sanitation and hygiene, the provision of more and better trained medical personnel at all levels. Regular orientation program of the primary care physician is mostly needed so that they can take prompt measures as soon as any epidemic occurs. It was evident that because of the resurgence of malaria in Kolkata after so many years doctors were not prepared to handle the situation efficiently. Health statistics in respect of differences of sex, age, occupation and social and economic status will contribute significantly in knowing the extent of the problem. Doctors are required to report, but in many cases their report is found to be grossly incomplete. Thus dedicated leadership among the doctors are required so that they can persuade others in preventing epidemic situation.

Sewerage and drainage facilities should be provided simultaneously with fresh supplies. Inadequate maintenance of newly constructed water and sewerage system has frequently created further health hazards.

References

- Central Bureau of Health Intelligence (1991). *Health Statistics of India*, Ministry of Health, New Delhi.
- *Harrison's Principals of Internal Medicine*, (2001) E. D. Braunwald, *et al.* 15th Edition, Vol. I & II.
- Mukherjee, B. (1999) *Gramin Swasthya*, Pavlov Institute.
- Myrdal, Gunar, (1968) *Asian Drama*, Vol. III, Penguin Books.